More praise for The Sexual Male

"This book may well be the best source of analysis as to the physiology, pathology, and management of erectile function that I have found. . . . The refreshing approach used by the authors of interplaying urological knowledge and management with the psychologist's perspective lends great credibility to the book."
—Tom E. Nesbitt, Sr., M.D., past president, American Medical Association

"Without using murky scientific language, the authors give the reader a new way to see what is the particular solution that best suits his situation. In fact, this would be a good book to read before there is any 'situation' at all, because Milsten and Slowinsky show many ways to prevent or diminish sexual problems and include many answers to ordinary, but important questions."   —Pepper Schwartz, Ph.D., coauthor of *What I've Learned About Sex: Leading Educators, Therapists, and Researchers Share Their Secrets*

"What a splendid idea for a prominent urologist to team up with a knowledgeable psychologist and write a state-of-the-art account of sexual dysfunction and its remedies. This user-friendly book is a delight to read, and its messages are very clear, easily found, and readily understood. Therapists and patients will find this book extremely beneficial."
—Arnold A. Lazarus, Ph.D.,
Distinguished Professor of Psychology Emeritus, Rutgers University

"*The Sexual Male* addresses many aspects of male sexual dysfunction in a scientific fashion, and manages to do so with a logical and practical viewpoint, interspersed with humor and personal philosophy."
—Alan J. Wein, M.D., professor and chair,
Division of Urology, University of Pennsylvania

"An engaging, comprehensive book about sexuality that has it all, from a clear explanation of the way the body works to the impact of the many psychological subtleties that influence how we behave and function sexually. It is unusual for books to include suggestions for self-evaluation and maintaining sexual health, yet these authors do this well."
—Derek C. Polonsky, M.D., Department of Psychiatry,
Harvard Medical School, and author of *Talking About Sex*

"Men (and women) trying to understand the causes and treatments of erection difficulties will welcome *The Sexual Male*. Broad coverage and clear presentation of important facts make this a useful resource."
—David Schnarch, Ph.D., author of *Passionate Marriage*

THE
SEXUAL
MALE

PROBLEMS
— AND —
SOLUTIONS

RICHARD MILSTEN, M.D.
AND JULIAN SLOWINSKI, PSY.D.

W. W. Norton & Company   New York • London

3 7834 00123387 2

To our patients who over the last thirty years
have allowed us to help them and taught us so much

Richard Milsten, M.D.
Medical Director
Center for Sexual Health

Julian Slowinski, Psy.D.
Senior Clinical Psychologist
Pennsylvania Hospital

For information about permission to reproduce selections from this book,
write to Permissions, W. W. Norton & Company, Inc., 500 Fifth Avenue,
New York, NY 10110

The text of this book is composed in Joanna and Cheltenham, with the display
set in Frutiger
Desktop composition by Thomas O. Ernst
Manufacturing by The Maple-Vail Book Manufacturing Group
Book design by Dana Sloan

Library of Congress Cataloging-In-Publication Data

Milsten, Richard.
    The sexual male: problems and solutions / Richard Milsten and
Julian Slowinski.
            p.   cm.
        Includes bibliographical references and index.
        ISBN 0-393-04740-7
        1. Impotence—Popular works. I. Slowinski, Julian W. II. Title.
RC889.M553   1999
616.6'92—dc21
                                                            99-17523
                                                            CIP

ISBN 0-393-32127-4 pbk.

W. W. Norton & Company, Inc.
500 Fifth Avenue, New York, N.Y. 10110
www.wwnorton.com

W. W. Norton & Company Ltd.
Castle House, 75/76 Wells Street, London W1T 3QT

2 3 4 5 6 7 8 9 0

ACKNOWLEDGMENTS

Our special thanks to Barbara J. Morgan, whose guidance and wise counsel are reflected throughout this book.

The thoughts of an author have to be transposed to paper. I would like to thank Sandie Nelson and Lisa McCammitt—two masters of the keyboard.
—*Richard Milsten, M.D.*

With gratitude to colleagues Dianne Gwynne Berger, Derek Polonsky, and Miki Wieder, whom I could count on to provide insightful comments on the text. A special thanks to Harold Lief, a friend and mentor throughout the years, whose clinical perspectives have greatly shaped the thinking behind the book.
—*Julian Slowinski, Psy.D.*

CONTENTS

FOREWORD

Dramatic changes have occurred in society's views of male sexuality since the advent of Viagra. This revolutionary new drug for the treatment of male erectile dysfunction broke all new drug sales records and became a household word in less than three months after its approval in March 1998. Viagra has brought the topic of male sexual dysfunction out of the closet as never before, and has led millions of men (and their sexual partners) to seek help for the problem. Despite the enormous numbers of men who have sought professional help in recent months, current estimates suggest that more than three-quarters of the men who have the problem have yet to address it. There is still much ignorance and anxiety surrounding the topic of male sexual dysfunction, in spite of the barrage of media coverage. And despite Viagra's effectiveness in alleviating symptoms of erectile dysfunction, it is not a panacea for all sexual or relationship problems.

In this highly readable and state-of-the-art guide to the topic, Milsten and Slowinski have provided readers—both men and women—with the latest information on medical causes and treatments for sexual dysfunction. Erection difficulties can be caused by many factors, and both physical and mental factors can play an important role. Few books provide such a broad and well-balanced discussion of the causes of sexual dysfunction and of the impact of the problem on individuals and their partner relationships. Both authors have extensive experience in helping men and their partners to cope with sexual difficulties, and the book is enriched by their clinical expertise and depth of understanding. The combined perspectives of the urologist and psychologist also provide a uniquely balanced approach to the subject matter at hand.

Perhaps the most valuable aspect of the book, however, is its explanation of the confusing array of new treatment options and alternatives. Who should take Viagra and what are the risks involved? Are there other oral medications available? Do penile injections still have a role to play? How do vacuum erection devices work, and who are they designed for? Is penile surgery a viable option, and can it be combined with medical treatments? These are only a few of the many treatment questions that this book addresses. In each case, the authors provide thorough, detailed, and up-to-date information for their readers. A thoughtful discussion of the advantages and disadvantages of each treatment is offered, which will be of great value to readers facing a choice between treatment options. The book is especially helpful in discussing the implications of treatment—what treatments can and can't do, and how to avoid disappointments.

In short, Milsten and Slowinski have broken new ground in their approach to the subject of male sexual dysfunction. This is one of the most thoughtful and intelligent books on the topic, and it will be an invaluable resource to the many men and women who are coping with sexual dysfunction and its consequences. I recommend it highly.

Raymond C. Rosen, Ph.D.
Co-Director, Center for Sexual and Marital Health
Robert Wood Johnson Medical School
Former President, International Academy of Sex Research

PREFACE

U nless you have recently been living on a different planet, you are aware of the increased attention being paid to the problem of impotence. This is primarily the result of the introduction of the first oral agent, Viagra, approved for use by the FDA, on March 27, 1998. Since this pill has become available, it has been commonplace for newspaper and magazine articles and radio and television shows to discuss this subject. Public awareness is at an all-time high.

We have taken a unique approach to provide you with the latest scientific information in an easily understandable manner, focusing on the causes of impotence, appropriate steps to diagnosis, and treatment options. The material represents the combined efforts and thoughts of both a urologist and a psychologist, because problems of impotence involve both specialties. Starting with the "basics," we will look at the history of impotence and the mechanics of how erections occur. The psychological and physical causes of impotence will be outlined, with emphasis on those that are most common. You will learn how to evaluate your own problem and where to seek help. The latest forms of treatment will be discussed, and you will learn the advantages and disadvantages of each. Topics of special interest, including sexual activity in patients with heart disease, whether or not bike riding will cause impotence, and whether there is a "male menopause," will be reviewed.

A special section on women's issues is included, since partners of impotent males may be affected. In addition, the question of impotence in the female will be brought into focus.

Impotence can be a problem for bisexual and gay men as well as straight men. For simplicity's sake, this book always refers to a man's partner as female, but for the most part the information it contains is just as applicable to gay men and their partners.

While other material written on this topic has focused primarily on treatment for impotence, we have chosen to emphasize how impotence may be *prevented*. The key to enjoying sex in your later years is outlined. How sexual activity correlates with increased longevity is spelled out.

The information in this book is intended not only for those males and their partners who are currently having difficulty with sexual functioning, but also for those who are presently enjoying a normal sex life. All males should be aware of the sexual problems they may encounter, and their partners should acquaint themselves with the causes of these problems so that they can either help to avert them or assist their male partner when difficulty occurs.

Couples who are involved in a sexual crisis should not ignore it, deny it, or hope that it will disappear by itself, because it rarely does. Nor should they assume that there is no remedy for their particular problem. On the contrary, most forms of sexual inadequacy can be dealt with. The key to the solution is knowledge. It is the goal of this book to offer advice on how to prevent impotence and to provide information in the hope that affected couples will understand how to begin making their sexual lives happier, more rewarding, and crisis-free.

A NOTE ON
THE PAPERBACK EDITION

Exciting advances in the treatment of erectile dysfunction continue to emerge. A second oral medication may promise help to many men. Apomorphine SL (trade name: Uprima, from TAP Pharmaceutical) facilitates erections through its action on the central nervous system by stimulating the "erection center" in the brain. Despite its chemical name, it is not an opiate. The tablet is placed under the tongue and allowed to dissolve. The time to erection is approximately fifteen to twenty-five minutes and the window for sexual activity is about two hours. The medication comes in varying strengths and adjustment by a physician is necessary. Patients report a success rate ranging between 45 and 60 percent depending upon dosage. As with all medications, certain side effects may occur. Nausea was reported by 17 percent of patients although more than half of these men described the side effect as "mild." Approximately 8 percent of patients reported feeling dizzy and the same percentage reported yawning. Many patients did not note these problems after taking the pill the first time.

A very promising cream that can be applied directly to the penis is undergoing clinical trials at the time of this writing. It contains a chemical (alprostadil) that is known to produce erections. This is similar to the agent that can be used for self-administered injections into the penis and is also the active ingredient in the pellet that is inserted into the opening of the penis (see Chapter 13). It has been combined with another chemical that allows penetration through the skin and into the erection compartments of the penis. The cream would have the advantage of being able to be used as a part of foreplay. However, an obvious concern is whether it will be absorbed in significant amounts through the wall of the vagina and cause effects in the female. Testing is being carried out by MacroChem Corporation and we are eager to see the results.

Female sexual functioning is also rapidly becoming an area of investigation for sex researchers. Sexual scientists realize that traditional models of human sexual response do not always directly apply to the special circumstances of women. There is a growing appreciation that the definition of sexual dysfunction for women is too broad. For example, the current definition includes interpersonal problems based on the partner's dissatisfaction even though the woman herself may not be experiencing subjective distress. Research is also underway to determine whether medications that have been developed to treat male sexual problems may also assist women to enjoy better sexual health.

LET'S BEGIN WITH WITH
WITH
THE BASICS

1

INTRODUCTION

Man can endure earthquake, epidemic, dreadful
disease, every form of spiritual torment; But the
most dreadful tragedy that can befall him is, and
will remain, the tragedy of the bedroom.

—*Tolstoy*

Key Points:

- Impotence affects twenty to thirty million men in the United
  States.
- An equal number of partners may be affected.
- Only a small percentage of males receive treatment.
- Impotence is not caused by aging alone.
- Impotence is treatable in virtually all cases and preventable in
  most.
- Impotence is no longer a taboo subject.
- As men live longer and boys experience sex at an earlier age, the
  problem assumes more and more importance.
- It is better to *prevent* impotence than to have to treat it—even
  with pills.

Most normal males, at sometime in their lives, will find themselves
unable to have an erection. This problem is not confined to the middle-
aged and the elderly but also happens to teenagers and males in their
twenties and thirties. For some men this condition develops suddenly

and is transient, but for others it may come on gradually and persist as a chronic problem.

Men whose sexual performance has been successful for years may one day find themselves unable to achieve an erection. This has been experienced even by males who have regarded themselves as marathon bedroom performers. Impotence, the consistent inability to attain and maintain an erection for satisfactory sexual performance, is one of the most common maladies in the United States for which treatment is available but not received. It is estimated that 20 to 30 million men in the United States suffer from erectile problems, yet only 5 to 10 percent seek treatment.

While the problem is, as one would expect, most common in middle-aged and older males, young men also have cause for concern. Even teenagers may suffer from impotence. (A recent study revealed that by age fifteen, approximately 27 percent of boys have already had sexual intercourse, and by age eighteen, the figure reaches almost 70 percent.)

In this country, where the standards of living and education are among the highest in the world, we are grossly ignorant about many areas of sexual functioning. Despite recent advances in understanding the physiology of the human sexual response, the average male and female know very little about the cause and effect of a male's inadequate sexual performance. We pride ourselves on caring for our newborn and on educating our children both at school and at home. We instruct them on what to eat and what clothes to wear, and we assist them in getting along with their peers. As children become teenagers, we assign them more and more responsibility in order to ensure their smooth transition into adulthood. We provide them with instruction on how to drive a car and how to become competent in various sports. Sex education classes are now fairly common at the high school and college level. Students are taught human anatomy and the mechanics of sexual functioning. But with rare exceptions, nowhere are they instructed on aspects of sexual failure. Many are not aware that it can occur, and even those who are aware are likely to assume that it is something that will happen to someone else.

Impotence is an *equal opportunity disease* not limited to any particular race, socioeconomic level, occupation, marital status, or religious belief. Democrat or Republican, any man is vulnerable! And when one considers that an impotent male's partner may be negatively affected, the magnitude of the problem doubles.

The good news for men who have the problem: it is treatable. The good news for men who have not yet experienced impotence: it is largely preventable.

Fortunately the topic of sexual dysfunction is no longer a taboo subject. Impotence is "out of the closet" and the subject continues to surface in books, lectures, and television talk shows.

The medical profession, recognizing that impotence affects between twenty and thirty million men in the United States, anticipated the importance of this topic. In December 1992, the National Institutes of Health issued a "Consensus Statement" dealing with this topic. Here are several of the panel's conclusions:

1. The likelihood of impotence increases with age but is not an inevitable consequence of aging.
2. Patients' embarrassment and the reluctance of both patients and health care providers to discuss sexual matters candidly contributes to underdiagnosis of impotence.
3. Impotence can be successfully managed with properly selected therapy.
4. Education of health care providers and the public on aspects of human sexuality is essential.
5. Impotence is an important public health problem that deserves increased support for basic investigation and applied research.

For patients considering treatment for impotence, there are four facts that should encourage them to seek help. First, there has been a vast amount of progress made in understanding the physiology and biochemistry of erections. Second, physicians, psychologists, and sex therapists are now better trained than ever before. Third, new treatments are now available, some of which are minimally invasive. Fourth, virtually every male suffering from impotence can resume a sexual relationship!

Impotence is best regarded as a "couples problem." While impotence may be catastrophic to the male, the difficulties that the female partner encounters should not be underestimated. A very solid relationship may be threatened or destroyed. The woman who does not understand her partner's "ups and downs" may become confused and uncertain, and may experience frustration, guilt, or anger. For younger women, the problem may be a "relationship breaker."

The introduction of Viagra provides hope to nearly all impotent males and treatment for a great many. (Other oral medications such as phentolamine and apomorphine await FDA approval.) However, major issues still need to be addressed. What is the underlying cause of the impotence—is it perhaps undiagnosed diabetes, narrowing of arteries, or another serious problem? What about interaction with one's partner? Is impotence really a reflection of a poor or deteriorating relationship?

In addition, not every impotent male can take "the pill." It cannot be used by anyone taking medications containing nitrates. And while it will help the majority of patients, millions of men will need to seek another avenue of treatment.

Most important, *PREVENTION* is preferable to any form of treatment.

Three critical facts about impotence underlie this book. The first is that many cases of impotence can be prevented through lifestyle changes, good medical care, better understanding, and psychological adjustments. The second is that impotence is not the inevitable consequence of aging. The third is that when problems with erections do occur, solutions, either medical or psychological, can be found for nearly every case. Very few have to resign themselves and conclude, "Well, I'll just have to live with it." The path to sexual health lies ahead.

It is our belief that:

> - *Wellness* is better than *illness*!
> - *Prevention* is better than *treatment*!
> - *Treatment* is better than *suffering*!

2

A LOOK AT THE PAST

Not to know what has been transacted in former
times is to continue always as a child.

—*Cicero*

Key Points:

- Impotence is not a new problem. It has always been a topic of
  concern.
- Over the centuries, many forms of treatment have been recommended—few of which are accepted methods today.
- Studies of the mechanism of erection have accelerated dramatically over the past twenty years.
- A better understanding of how erections occur has opened the
  door to new, minimally invasive treatment options.

The problem of impotence is age-old. It is well documented in history. Sexual anxiety in childhood as a cause of impotence in adult life
was recorded in Greek mythology. King Phylacus asked his physician,
Melampus, to cure his son, Iphiculs, who was suffering from impotence. Melampus discovered that in childhood Iphiculs had seen his
father brandishing a bloodstained gelding knife. He became terrified
that he was going to be castrated, and it was this fright that allegedly
accounted for his impotence in later years. By carefully pointing out
how his fear had developed, Melampus was able to cure Iphiculs of his
impotence.

A passage from Genesis (20:1) has been interpreted by some as a description of how Abimelech became impotent as divine punishment for taking Abraham's wife: "But God came to Abimelech in a dream by night and said to him, behold, thou art a dead man, for the woman which thou has taken; for she is a man's wife."

The preoccupation of man with sexual potency and his fear of impotence is evident in literature and mythology throughout the centuries. For the ancients the potency of the king was believed to affect the success of the harvest and well-being of the people. Impotence was often seen as resulting from a divine curse or the result of bewitchment called down by a vengeful enemy.

Beginning in the Middle Ages and for many years thereafter, impotence was believed to result from a curse inflicted by witches. A dramatic example of this concerns Don Carlos (1661–1700), who was the last of the Spanish Hapsburgs. He failed to give Spain an heir; this later led to the War of the Spanish Succession. Don Carlos was described as physically weak and of limited mental ability as a result of many generations of inbreeding. Despite two marriages, he was unable to produce the vitally needed heir to assure continuation of his family line. It was believed that he was impotent. Exorcisms were performed, but his impotence persisted to the end of his life. When he died, so did the Spanish Hapsburgs.

In the Middle Ages, those practicing witchcraft believed that impotence could be produced by tying knots in a cord or strip of leather and then hiding the knotted piece. This practice was known as ligature, and the affected party supposedly remained impotent until the cord was found and untied.

Witchcraft and impotence played a significant role in the history of several western nations. King James I of England wrote the treatise *Daemonologie* on the subject. James intervened in the trial in which the Countess of Essex attempted to divorce her husband on the grounds of impotence.

Some important literary figures were afflicted with sexual difficulties. For instance, George Bernard Shaw's sexual life is controversial. While some believe he was promiscuous, others believe he was impotent. Some have attributed the conjectured impotence to homosexual tendencies that caused Shaw sexual anxiety. His own marriage was described as one of "contractual sexlessness."

Rousseau related an episode of impotence that occurred when he was with an attractive prostitute. "Suddenly, instead of the fire that devoured me, I felt a deathly cold flow through my veins; my legs trembled; I sat down on the point of fainting and wept like a child."

Twenty-three hundred years ago, Hippocrates noted that a preoccupation with business as well as a lack of female attractiveness could cause impotence. And the Hindus warned that impotence could follow an encounter with a female a man found distasteful.

The *Malleus Maleficarum*, a manual dealing with witchcraft published in 1488, discussed the causes and treatment of impotence. Remedies included the use of splints and special herbs.

The reticence about discussing sexual topics in Victorian times rendered impotence an unlikely topic in literature, and the condition was only hinted at obliquely. For example, George Elliot's *Middlemarch* recalls the impending marriage between the elderly former clergyman Edward Casubon and the young and attractive Dorthea Brooke with the comment: "Good God! It is horrible. He is no better than a mummy. For this marriage to Casubon is as good as going into a nunnery."

While the fear of impotence plagues the ordinary man, biographers point out that notable figures such as D. H. Lawrence, King Richard I, Louis XVI, Napoleon, and Edgar Allan Poe were troubled with impotence at some time in their lives for various reasons. One theory held is that sexual continence is directly related to artistic creativity and dedication to one's profession. Names such as Chekhov, Flaubert, Beethoven, Lamb, and Ruskin, as well as celibate clergymen, bear witness to this opinion.

The concern and preoccupation with male potency has been a subject for the arts and a private worry of the common man. The frequency of impotence as a theme has reached to the point where one review of Edward Albee's *Who's Afraid of Virginia Woolf* stated: "It also dwells on impotence, a long established Broadway theme that has lately hardened into an obsession. No serious play is complete without it."

As for worries of the "man in the street," Lawrence Durrell reminds us of this common concern in his novel *Balthazar* with the words of the

Frenchman Pombal: "His only preoccupation is with losing his job or being impotent: the national worry of every Frenchman since Jean-Jacques."

Even today an unconsummated marriage due to impotence can be the cause for annulment of a marriage in the Roman Catholic Church. Impotence that is known to preexist marriage is an impediment to the reception of the sacrament of marriage in the Catholic Church.

Many societies devised their own unique methods of treating impotence. In Europe, "phallic foods" were once popular; these included fresh eggs, lobsters, leguminous plants, French beans, and oysters. Years ago, Egyptians regarded the crocodile's penis as a symbol of virility. Some actually ate the crocodile's penis in order to increase their potency.

Treatments that were in vogue only forty years ago now seem rather curious. Metal rods were either heated or cooled and then passed into the penis in order to alleviate any inflammation therein. Another form of therapy consisted of electrical shocks to the testicles. Some doctors advocated an operation to tighten the muscles beneath the scrotum, which were considered to be weak. A most interesting apparatus was the penile splint. This peculiar-looking device allowed the male to penetrate the female even when his penis was soft.

From a historical viewpoint, enormous strides have been made in the treatment of erectile insufficiency, and these will be covered later. It is of interest, however, to look to the researchers of the past. The work of Ancel and Bouin in France in the early 1900s and that of Steinach in the 1920s suggested that vasectomy promoted sexual rejuvenation. In 1936, Niehans noted the positive effects of this procedure in correcting impotence. In 1918, Voronoff, a Parisian, declared that youth could be restored by transplanting a portion of monkey testicles into man. That same year, Lespianasse, a professor of genitourinary surgery at Northwestern University, treated male impotence by implanting slices of human testicles taken from fresh cadavers into a small incision made in the abdomen of the sexually inadequate male.

Stanley, a physician working with a captive population at San Quentin Prison in California, published a paper in 1922 citing a thousand testicular implant surgical procedures that had been performed on 656 patients. Unlike Lespianasse, who used human testicular tissue, Stanley chose the testicles of goats, rams, boars, and deer. The testicles from these animals were cut into strips with a knife in sizes suitable for the filling of a pressure syringe. The testicular substance was then injected by force underneath the skin of the abdomen. Stanley noted no significant difference in the effects produced by the testicular material taken from the various animals. Today, testicular implantation, using either human material or material obtained from animals, is not considered a valid procedure.

Evidence of the increasing interest in the scientific study of impotence and other sexual problems is seen in medical textbooks. Campbell's textbook of urology has been a bible for the urologist for many years. In the third edition, published in 1970, approximately one page is devoted to impotence and four pages to masturbation. Premature ejaculation is not even discussed. In the fifth edition of this text, published in 1986, the topic of premature ejaculation is given only four sentences. In the sixth edition of Campbell's *Urology*, published in 1992, more than fifty pages are devoted to the problems of impotence. The problem of premature ejaculation is given a single page.

An important period is unfolding in the history of impotence. Our knowledge of the causes of and the appropriate treatment for erectile insufficiency is increasing exponentially. As knowledge continues to accelerate, a new understanding of how an erection occurs has led to a variety of simpler and more acceptable treatments.

3

WHAT IS IMPOTENCE?

Definitions might be good things if only we did not
employ words in making them.

—*Rousseau*

Key Points:

- Impotence is the consistent inability to attain or sustain an
  erection sufficient for satisfactory sexual performance.
- Impotence is not the same problem as sterility, loss of libido
  (sex drive), or premature ejaculation.
- In this text, the terms "erectile insufficiency", "erectile dysfunction," and "impotence" will be used interchangeably.

Impotence is the inability to attain or sustain an erection sufficient for satisfactory sexual performance. Impotence may take many
forms. For example, a male may be able to achieve an erection and
begin intercourse, but the penis may become soft before completion
of the act.

There is a movement in medical circles to rename impotence "erectile insufficiency." This is consistent with medical terminology used to
designate problems in other organs, such as liver failure (hepatic insufficiency), heart failure (cardiac insufficiency), kidney failure (renal insufficiency), and failure of the lungs (pulmonary insufficiency). Another
term sometimes used to describe impotence is "erectile dysfunction." In
this book, all three terms will be used and are considered synonymous.

This is in conformity with other written information on the subject as well as terminology used in the media.

F.D., a fifty-year-old attorney, noticed a change in his sexual ability approximately three months before seeking medical attention. His past history was not unusual, and he had not experienced prior difficulties with intercourse. However, recently he had noticed that while his erections started out in a normal fashion, the penis seemed to soften upon attempted insertion into the vagina. Initially, he attributed this to a state of physical fatigue, but when it occurred persistently, he sought advice. His female partner was very aware of the difficulty because the sexual act did not last long enough for her to have an orgasm.

Certain males may be able to achieve an erection only when gazing at pornographic material or in complete privacy. However, these individuals cannot perform with a female partner.

A.G., a thirty-one-year-old male, had been raised in a strict religious setting in which sexual activities were frowned upon. Masturbation was not acceptable in his society. He related to his physician that he had no trouble achieving an erection when he saw pornographic material either in a magazine or a movie, but that he had not been able to consummate his recent marriage because of failure to get a sufficient erection.

Some men can function sexually with a prostitute or other women for whom they have no emotional feelings but find themselves impotent with a woman for whom they truly care.

S.R., a forty-seven-year-old male, never married, had recently begun dating an attractive woman who worked in his office. He respected her greatly, and they developed a close emotional relationship. He regarded her as a very special person. His sexual history was normal, and on one occasion, five years earlier, he had gotten a woman pregnant and she had had an abortion. On his first occasion in bed with his new female companion, he could not achieve an erection. Despite her patience and encouragement, intercourse did not occur.

Certain males can perform only if they fantasize that they are with a different woman.

> *D.M., a thirty-eight-year-old male, had been married for seven years and was the father of two children. Recently his sexual interest in his wife had seemed to decline, and intercourse usually occurred only if she initiated it. Erections became increasingly difficult to attain and maintain until it reached the point where D.M. would close his eyes during intercourse and imagine that he was in the arms of his secretary.*

Some males cannot understand why sometimes they are able to perform well sexually, yet at other times are unable to perform at all.

> *M.F., a forty-four-year-old male, directed a highly successful business that he had founded. He had his emotional ups and downs, which seemed to be connected with how well his business was running. He enjoyed sexual activity, and he and his wife had intercourse two or three times a week. After a six-week period in which he was unable to achieve an erection, he sought medical attention. During this same period of time, he was in the midst of a lawsuit that threatened his company's financial position.*

Some individuals who have repeatedly failed to get an erection despite the most opportune circumstances declare that they are not really interested in sex and won't try again.

> *B.F., a sixty-one-year-old executive, was forced by his female partner to see a physician because of impotence. When they were interviewed, the woman complained that her partner was not interested in sex at all. In private, B.F. disclosed that he had attempted intercourse with a young secretary from his office and with another woman whom he had met at a recent business convention. Both of these women were unusually attractive and most receptive to his advances. Yet he had been unable to achieve an erection with either of them. He had now failed with three different women in a very short period of time. His sexual drive had waned, and he expressed a general disinterest in sexual activity.*

All of the above are examples of impotence. While some men can't get an erection, others complain of not being able to maintain one long enough to complete sexual activity. Certain men can function sexually only with some women, but not with others. Some can achieve an erection and ejaculate through self-stimulation, but not with a female partner. Despite some differences, all of the above problems are variations on a common theme—a lack of satisfactory erections.

Medical authorities divide impotence into primary and secondary forms. Primary impotence refers to the rare male who has never in his life had an erection sufficient for sexual performance. In secondary impotence, which comprises the vast majority of cases, a male has had erections and engaged in successful intercourse in the past but currently his erectile ability is significantly reduced or absent.

In order to understand disorders of male sexual function, certain other terms need to be defined. "Ejaculation" refers to the projection of semen. This is caused by contraction of muscular tissue within the penis and pelvis. "Orgasm" occurs at the culmination of the sexual act and is a pleasurable sensation representing both physical and psychological response to ejaculation.

Disorders of ejaculation, including uncontrollable (premature) ejaculation and failure to ejaculate, are not, strictly speaking, a part of impotence, but either of these conditions represents inadequate sexual performance and may lead to an impotent state.

"Impotence" and "sterility" are commonly confused terms. Sterility is the inability to have children and is often due to a lack of production of a sufficient number of normal living sperm. A sterile man may be able to have good erections. An impotent man, on the other hand, may produce sperm of normal quality but not be able to impregnate his partner because he cannot achieve an erection sufficiently strong to permit successful intercourse.

There is another crisis that many impotent men experience—loss of libido. Loss of libido is a decline in sexual interest or urge—a dwindling sex drive. When impotent males are asked to list other sexual problems, this is one of the most often cited. The fact is that a decrease in libido may occur as a consequence of impotence or it may precede the onset of erectile difficulties. On the surface, it is easy to understand how a man who cannot achieve an erection sufficient for intercourse may, after a period of time, lose interest. Whether this is a defense mechanism may be debated.

It is more common for a loss of libido to follow the onset of impotence than to precede it. In either instance, it may be a cause of great concern to the male. He may wonder if it is another sign of a generalized deterioration.

4

UNDERSTANDING ERECTIONS

There may be some things better than sex, and
some things may be worse, but there is nothing
exactly like it.

—*W. C. Fields*

Key Points:

- An erection may be caused by physical or mental stimulation.
- An erection is due to the inflow and storage of blood in the penis.
- Erections are dependent upon the normal function of the vascular and nervous systems.
- The chemical transmitters that cause an erection have recently been identified, opening the door for the development of oral medication to treat impotence.
- Stages of the normal sexual response from arousal to orgasm are now understood, and each has its own characteristics.

In order to understand impotence, it is necessary to understand the mechanism of erections.

An erection is a reflex involving little voluntary control. A man unfortunately cannot command himself to have an erection. On the other hand, sometimes an erection occurs at an inopportune time;

nearly every man at one time or another has had to button his raincoat, turn over onto his belly at the beach, or take other action in order to conceal an erection.

One of the major contributions of William H. Masters and Virginia E. Johnson has been to detail the physiology of the male sexual response. Their observations were based on studying more than three hundred men whose ages ranged from the early twenties to the late eighties and who participated in a total of more than 2,500 sexual encounters. Masters and Johnson noted four phases of sexual response. In the "excitement phase," blood rushes into the penis faster than it is drained away, so that an erection occurs. The rigidity of the penis thus comes from blood that circulates throughout the body being directed into the erectile tissue of the penis (the corpora cavernosa). This tissue is like a sponge that accepts blood and becomes very firm. Routing the blood to the penis requires a normal nervous system. With sexual excitement, the testicles draw upward into the scrotum and the opening at the end of the penis begins to enlarge. In some men, the nipples become firm and erect. The muscles of the legs and arms may become tense, and the rate of breathing increases.

In the second phase of sexual response, the "plateau phase," the head of the penis, known as the glans, increases in diameter. The testicles are maximally elevated within the scrotum. Muscular tension is increased and there is involuntary contraction of the facial muscles, so that the male actually begins to frown. A fine red rash may develop over the neck, face, and upper chest. A few drops of seminal fluid may be released from the end of the penis.

During the third phase, the "orgasmic phase," the male experiences a feeling that ejaculation is imminent and inevitable. At this time, the secretions from several glands, including the testicles and prostate, are deposited in the urethra. This results in the man's experiencing a sensation that semen is about to be released. As the muscles of the urethra and penis contract, the opening to the bladder closes, so that the seminal fluid mixed with sperm shoots forth from the penis. A volume of one to five cubic centimeters (about a teaspoon) is ejected one to two feet out of the end of the penis. The rate of breathing may increase to more than thirty breaths per minute. The mouth usually remains open. The heart rate shoots up to between 100 and 180 beats per minute, and the blood pressure may rise significantly. At the time of orgasm there may be involuntary contraction of the muscles of the legs, buttocks, and feet.

It has often been assumed that the male's perception of orgasm is different from the female's. However, one study indicates that the written descriptions of orgasm are very similar for both sexes. When these descriptions were studied by physicians, psychologists, and medical students, not one expert could tell which had been written by men and which by women. Here are some of them:

A sudden feeling of light-headedness followed by an intense feeling of relief and elation. A rush. Intense muscular spasms of the whole body. Sense of euphoria followed by deep peace and relaxation.

Feels like tension building up until you think it can't build up any more, then release. The orgasm is both the highest point of tension and the release almost at the same time. Also feeling contractions in the genitals. Tingling all over.

Obviously, we can't explain what it feels "like" because it feels "like" nothing else in human experience. A poetic description may well describe the emotions that go with it, but the physical "feeling" can only be described with very weak mechanical terminology. It is a release that occurs after a period of manipulation has sufficiently enabled internal, highly involuntary spasms that are pleasurable due to your complete involuntary control (no control). It's like shooting junk on a sunny day in a big, green, open field.

I really think it defies description by words. Combination of waves of very pleasurable sensations and mounting of tensions culminating in a fantastic sensation and release of tension.

Orgasm gives me a feeling of unobstructed intensity of satisfaction. Accompanied with the emotional feeling and love one has for another, the reality of the sex drive, and our culturally conditioned status on sex, an orgasm is the only experience that sends my body and mind into a state of beautiful oblivion.

Tension builds to an extremely high level—muscles are tense, etc. There is a sudden expanding feeling in the pelvis and muscle spasms throughout the body followed by release of tension. Muscles relax and consciousness returns.

A building of tension, sometimes, and frustration until the climax. A tightening inside, palpitating rhythm, explosion, and warmth and peace.

A feeling where nothing much else enters the mind other than that which relates to the present, oh sooo enjoyable and fulfilling sensation. It's like jumping into a cool swimming pool after hours of sweating turmoil. "Ahhh! Relief!" What a great feeling it was, so ecstatically wild and all right!

A feeling of intense physical and mental satisfaction. The height of a sexual encounter. Words can hardly describe a feeling so great.

The fourth phase of sexual response described by Masters and Johnson is called "resolution." Following ejaculation, the penis softens as blood drains out of it. During that time, a male cannot achieve another erection despite the most vigorous stimulation. The length of this period varies from man to man. Hence the female should expect and the male accept the fact that he may not be able to perform again for a certain amount of time. There is no doubt that this period increases with age, and that older individuals will require more time than younger ones to achieve the next erection.

During resolution, the scrotum relaxes and the testicles descend. The skin flush disappears, and the man may perspire lightly, particularly on the palms and soles.

During the 1970s the thinking of the experts was that the erection process was controlled by valvelike structures called "polsters." These were thought to be muscle cells in the walls of the blood vessels supplying the penis. In the nonerect state the polsters in the arteries were thought to be contracted. Polsters in the veins were thought to be relaxed. The result was that blood was shunted away from the erectile tissue of the penis. At the time of erection, the opposite was thought to occur. The polsters in the arteries relaxed and those in the veins contracted. This permitted blood to flow into the penis and restricted its outflow, thus resulting in an erection.

As knowledge increased, it was learned that the polsters were really artifacts of atherosclerotic plaques and did not function as specialized valves. Supporting evidence was that polsters were not present in blood vessels of young males.

Enormous strides have been made in the past two decades in understanding the mechanism of erections. A successful erection depends upon the inflow into and storage of blood in the erectile compartments within the penis. If things are functioning properly, blood enters the penis faster than it drains and hence there is a buildup of pressure, as in a hydraulic system, and the penis becomes erect. (When the penis is not erect, it is stated to be in the "flaccid" state.) The penis becomes enlarged (tumescent) and finally rigid (erect). Normally the process of erection begins when the brain receives stimulation, which may be either physical (direct touching of the genitalia) or mental. Mental stimulation may be visual, auditory, olfactory, or tactile (touching).

The erectile tissue of the penis can be thought of as a spongelike material. With stimulation, the message is sent via nerve impulses that cause a relaxation of blood vessels in the spongy erectile tissue. At this point the penis begins to swell. As swelling increases, the spongy tissue presses against veins that would normally drain blood from the penis. With compression, the veins do not allow the blood to escape, and hence, as the erectile compartments continue to fill, the penis becomes rigid.

In the last decade, scientists have identified the chemicals within the body that are responsible for the relaxation of the erectile tissue that permits blood to build up until the penis is rigid. They are nitric oxide and cyclic guanosine monophosphate (cGMP).

The good news is that as investigators continue to unravel the physiological and biochemical pathways that lead to an erection, more opportunity exists for the pharmaceutical industry to offer treatment choices. In fact, it is this new understanding that has paved the way for the development of oral medication to treat problems of erectile insufficiency. (See Chapter 14.)

For those who wish a more detailed understanding of the penile anatomy and erectile function, the following section is provided. Those readers who are content with a more general understanding may want to skip ahead to Chapter 5.

ANATOMY OF THE PENIS

The erectile tissue of the penis may be thought of as three cylinders (Fig. 1). The two major cylinders, the corpora cavernosa, are located as paired structures in the top of the penis. The corpora spongiosum, located beneath the corpora cavernosum, is a single cylinder that surrounds the urethra, the tube through which urine passes. Inside each cylinder are smooth muscle fibers, blood, and nerves that form small compartments called "lacunar spaces." It is these spaces that fill with blood to create an erection. As these spaces distend, they compress

Figure 1 **Penile structures**

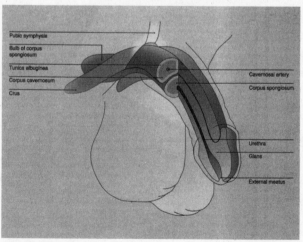

against the outside lining (the tunica albuginea) of the three corpora, which results in compression of the veins that drain the penis. Hence, blood accumulates and expansion and ultimately rigidity of the penis occur (Fig. 2).

As the blood vessels and lacunar spaces relax, blood flow increases until pressure inside the corpora reaches a point when the blood flow slows down dramatically. Following ejaculation, the muscles of the arteries and lacunar spaces contract and blood flow is thereby diminished, which decreases the pressure on the emissary veins, allowing blood to return to the general circulation. The end result is that the once rigid penis is now soft (flaccid).

BLOOD SUPPLY

How does the blood get to the penis? The artery to the penis (which arises from the internal pudendal artery, a branch of the hypogastric

Figure 2 **Penile blood supply**

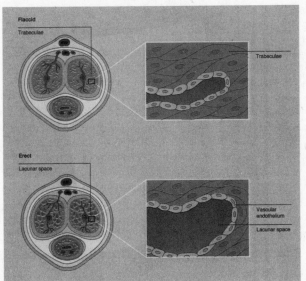

Figure 3 **Penile blood supply**

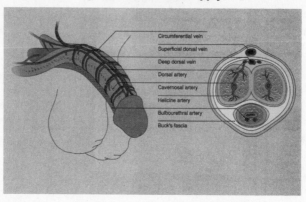

Circumferential vein
Superficial dorsal vein
Deep dorsal vein
Dorsal artery
Cavernosal artery
Helicine artery
Bulbourethral artery
Buck's fascia

artery) supplies branches to the erectile compartments of the corpora cavernosa and the corpus spongiosum. Within the corpora, the arteries divide into smaller branches called helicine arterioles (Fig. 3). It is these arteries that supply the blood to the lacunar spaces.

Blood entering the penis must be carried away and returned to the general circulation. The small veins that begin to drain each corpora are termed emissary veins. Ultimately these form a larger vein (the cavernosal vein), which then drains into a yet larger vein (the internal pudendal vein).

NERVE SUPPLY TO THE PENIS

The function of the smooth muscle and arteries and veins is under the control of nerve fibers (the autonomic nervous system, Fig. 4). Two different types of nerves activate and deactivate the erectile process. The sympathetic nervous system keeps the blood flow to the penis reduced and the lacunar spaces contracted (flaccid state). The parasympathetic nervous system is responsible for the opposite response, relaxation of the smooth muscle of the lacunar spaces and the blood vessels.

Erections that originate in the brain (in the thalamus and the medial preoptic areas) are called psychogenic erections. Such erections may be initiated by an erotic thought or auditory, tactile, olfactory, or visual stimuli, such as a titillating message whispered in the ear, a touch on

Figure 4 **Penile innervation**

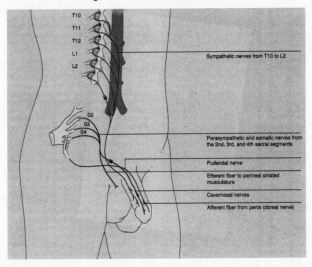

the skin, the smell of perfume, or an erotic picture. Erections may also be initiated by direct stimulation of the genitalia (reflexogenic erection), such as occurs during foreplay.

The nervous system is also responsible for the deposition and expulsion of semen from the urethra at the time of ejaculation. The sensation of orgasm is a complex psychophysiologic mechanism that has not yet been fully elucidated.

Nerve signals are relayed by chemicals called neurotransmitters. While many chemicals participate in the chain of events, two of the most important for erections are nitric oxide (NO) and cyclic guanosine monophosphate (cGMP).

We have made great strides in understanding erections, and the information gleaned from the laboratory is helping us in treating erectile failure.

UNDERSTANDING THE CAUSES
OF YOUR PROBLEM

5

PSYCHOLOGICAL CAUSES OF IMPOTENCE

What you discover on your own is always more
exciting than what someone else discovers for
you—it's like the difference between romantic love
and an arranged marriage.

—*Terrence Rafferty*

Key Points:

- Male sexual identity is closely tied to male self-identity.
- Our sexual scripts may determine both the cause of and the response to erectile problems. These sexual scripts are partly a product of our early learning experiences, including family attitudes about sexuality.
- Sexual problems are often rooted in the relationship between partners, including the level of trust and quality of intimacy. In many ways, the penis does not lie.
- Sexual problems often occur with new partners. It is important to make appropriate choices about when, where, and with whom to have sex.

Before we can talk about sexual health and prevention of sexual dysfunctions, we must first attempt to consider the causes that contribute to erectile problems. The potential causes are many. Some are self-evident, such as an episode of impotence caused by drinking too much alcohol. Other causes of erectile problems are deeper psychological issues that are often outside conscious awareness and may require more exploration to uncover. The task of understanding causes of impotence will be made easier if we continually keep in mind the emotional interplay that exists between the overall personal experience of the man, his relationship with his partner, and the situation or circumstances in which sexual activity occurs.

THE PERSON: WHO IS THIS MAN?

John was the eldest of three brothers raised in a Roman Catholic family. In his household, respect for rules and denial of self-interest were considered admirable virtues. Sex was not discussed at home, and his parents never showed overt signs of affection for each other in front of the boys. John's parochial school education had left him with a mild distrust of his sexual feelings. In fact, he felt guilty during his teenage years about his emerging sexual feelings and his occasional masturbation. He also felt guilty about his early attempts at sexual experimentation with girls in high school and college, even though he received peer support and encouragement for these sexual activities.

Then John met Carol. He really cared about her, and at first was refreshed by her openness about sexual matters. They eventually did have sex, and John was surprised to admit to himself that he enjoyed being sexual with Carol. But John soon began to grow uneasy about Carol's enjoyment of sex. She was obviously more comfortable with sex than he was. John felt confused and caught between his positive feelings for Carol and his growing sense of uneasiness about having sex with her. Was there something wrong with her because she liked sex so much? Was Carol, after all, "that kind of girl," one who enjoyed sex too much? Was she the kind that guys "really didn't marry"? She was too easy. As time went by, John grew more ambivalent about Carol and having sex with her. He actually began to have trouble getting or holding his erections. He refused to acknowledge that he was becoming overwhelmed with guilt about sex with Carol, and that his body was just reacting to those negative feelings. By this time, Carol was becoming displeased. Whenever she wanted to talk about it, John refused. They were going nowhere fast.

Like John, we all grew up somewhere, and usually in a family and community that helped form us and our understanding of life. In other words, we all have a developmental history that includes early experiences, which in many ways shaped attitudes toward matters of living. These attitudes in turn affected our own behavior and our view of the behavior of others. For example, growing up in a small rural town in close proximity to the family and local community provides a different life experience from growing up in an urban environment characterized by separation and anonymity. Despite these wide differences of life experience, people are all faced with the same developmental tasks of gaining a sense of self by going through the stages of childhood, teenage years, and adulthood. This sense of self, or self-identity, is the fruit of an ongoing process that, while it is lifelong, does lay its foundation in the early years of life and childhood. We relate to the world in terms of our self-identity. That is why, for example, a man who has erectile failure is vulnerable to experiencing some loss of self-esteem. His image of himself as a properly functioning sexual male is called into question by his failure to perform up to his own expectations. How a man feels about himself sexually, as a male, is a part of his sexual identity, and becomes part of how he views himself as a male, regardless of whether he is straight, gay, or bisexual. Men (and women) bring this sense of self to every personal interaction they engage in, especially sexual encounters. A great part of how we relate to others sexually is determined by what sex therapists have come to call a person's sexual script.

SEXUAL SCRIPT: WHAT IS IT?

Sex therapists borrowed the term "sexual script" from the observations of sociologists William Simon and John Gagnon. To understand our own sexual script—everyone has one—all we have to do is think of the range and repertoire of our sexual experiences, feelings, attitudes, and behaviors. A sexual script is the lens through which we view sexuality, our own and that of others. It becomes both a cause and an effect of our sexual experience. Our sexual script is reflected in what we do or do not do sexually. It determines how a couple negotiates sex in their shared sexual life. It is operating when we have our private opinions about the behavior of others. It is reflected in attitudes that range from bigotry to an "anything goes" attitude about sexuality. It is a reflection of our own personal psychology about sexuality in action.

In itself, sexual script is neither a good or bad thing—only our actions and intentions can make it so. It just is. However, our sexual script does determine how we allow ourselves to experience and act on our sexuality. A rigid or narrow sexual script not only limits our willingness to express and experience our sexuality, but in a relationship it can determine what happens between partners. Sexual difficulties between partners are often a reflection of their opposing sexual scripts. What may be "normal" behavior to one partner can be "perversion" to another. Understanding your sexual script can help you understand both the roots of impotence and the maintenance of sexual health. Let us explore the origins of our development of our attitudes towards sex, our bodies, and being in intimate relationships with others.

FAMILY VALUES ARE NOT ALWAYS HEALTHY

What kind of values and attitudes about sex did John learn at home? We can think back to our earliest memories about sex that we learned from our families. Many people say, "What memories? Sex was never discussed at home." If this was the case, an attitude of silence about sex usually implied either a negative message or a general sense of discomfort with the body and sexual feelings. Kids are perceptive and quickly understand what not to ask questions about at home. Herein lies the beginning of the great conspiracy of silence about sex. How many of us were taught sex-positive notions about the goodness and enjoyment of sexual pleasure? To have been exposed to sex-positive messages was a privilege.

Some of the messages youngsters receive vary according to ethnic group and degree of religious observance. Often the message young people get is deeply conflicted: "Sex is dirty. Save it for someone you love." While some ethnic heritages tend to celebrate the earthy joys of life and the acceptance of the range of human emotions, others tend to be closed to the expression and the experience of too much feeling. Yet, all people have a similar genetic and hormonal endowment that is destined to fulfill nature's sexual intentions. These strong sexual feelings are inborn in us whether we embrace and celebrate them or deny and struggle with them. Therapists refer to the "repression" of feelings as an unconscious action, while the term "suppression" refers to a conscious intention of putting away certain feelings that may make the person uncomfortable.

These mental mechanisms are not necessarily bad things. It is often appropriate to suppress sexual feelings. For example, we all know there are times when the prudent thing to do is to keep our mouth shut, especially about sexual comments. However, when it comes to a steady pattern of refusing to acknowledge or deal constructively with sexual feelings, the long-term result can be heightened feelings of shame, guilt, and anxiety. Given this background, it is not surprising that a man (or woman) might experience difficulty or even dysfunction in a future sexual situation. A good predictor of our comfort level of sexual functioning as an adult is how we emerge from our personal sexual development during our adolescence.

JUST WHAT IS SEXUAL DEVELOPMENT?

Sexual development in adolescence refers to more than just the sexual maturing of the body. Our development into sexual beings is the result of a process of many interactive events and experiences that shape and form us and eventually determine how we relate to each other as sexual persons. It is a process that sex therapists Philip and Lorna Sarrel refer to as sexual unfolding. One of the features of sexual unfolding is a growing sense of one's body that is realistic, well informed, and not confused by misinformation—a growing sense and comfortable acceptance of one's body. For boys, for example, the concern about the appearance and size of their penis could be an issue. Just as many women recall earlier anxiety about their developing breasts, men also are frequently not pleased with their penis.

How much is enough? Myths about size and potency are passed on from generation to generation and continue to do potential harm to the developing male sense of sexual adequacy. A male's sexual ignorance about the normal functioning of his own as well as the female body can be a significant cause of later sexual difficulties. Many men enter therapy with sexual problems only to find out that their difficulties are rooted in basic ignorance and misinformation about what to expect from their own body and that of their partners. Too many men expect themselves to be sexual athletes and have unrealistic beliefs. Do these same men worry that they cannot run the 100-yard dash at a world-class level, or for that matter, run it as well as when they were in high school? Of course not! Yet men frequently punish themselves for not living up to what is in fact an unrealistic sexual standard. They forget about real factors like individual differences between men and the effects of the aging process on overall bodily function. While they may accept the fact that they need to wear bifocals to assist their vision, they may be ignoring the fact that their aging penis may need more direct stimulation in order to achieve an erection. Gone is the instant erection of youth. What is so wrong with the assisted erection of middle age? When it comes to sex, ignorance is not always bliss!

Overcoming shame and guilt resulting from earlier messages about sexuality is a further task of development. Private sexual thoughts, feelings, and behaviors, such as masturbation, often present the adolescent with considerable conflict. These conflicts can be complicated by sex-negative messages from family or religious teachings. This may include issues related to questions about sexual orientation. If gay, the adolescent male has limited resources and role models available to him to answer his questions and quiet his confusion. Meeting and mastering these and other challenges are important for enjoying adult sexual health.

As a young person moves through early experiences with sexual partners, a healthy sense of the place of sex in his or her life should develop. This includes a growing ability to value one's sexuality as an act of intimacy with another, not just as a satisfaction of biological functioning. It includes practicing safe sex. It means emerging into adulthood with an appreciation of one's self as a sexual person, and with respect for the sexual rights of others, including the right not to engage in sexual activity.

Moving toward sexual maturity and adult sexual health involves putting together many pieces of a complex puzzle of life experiences. The successful completion of these developmental tasks that we have outlined can be complicated by other forces. For example, any sexual trauma, such as inappropriate or early exposure to sexual behavior or sexual violence or molestation, can contribute to later difficulties in adult sexual adjustment. Given the complexity of the factors involved in acquiring healthy sexual development, one wonders how many adults mastered the tasks of sexual unfolding as adolescents. Unfinished business with normal developmental issues can catch up with a man and may impact erectile functioning in his future sexual relationships.

PERSONALITY COUNTS

While certain mental disorders are frequently accompanied by erectile problems, the general population experiences more subtle, but nonetheless important, personality issues that can influence potency. There are personality styles and disorders that can contribute to erectile failure. Some conditions, such as depression, may tend to reduce a man's interest in sex. Other personality problems and conflicts are played out in the sexual relationship with the partner and may complicate the quality of intimacy. These can be underlying contributors to erectile failure. Even well-intended treatment can have negative sexual side effects. For example, certain antidepressant medications can further interfere with desire and the erectile process.

The existence of a manic state can also interfere with sexual functioning. Other men are chronic worriers. A preoccupation with perfection and performance can incline a man to worry about his sexual functioning to the point of contributing to erectile failure. Such men are prone to anticipatory and performance anxiety and can worry themselves into impotence. Their chronic anxiety prevents them from relaxing enough to tune in to and experience sexual cues that would ordinarily arouse them.

Some men play out their personality difficulties in the overall sexual relationship and can experience erectile failure as a consequence. The man who tends to deal with the world in a passive-aggressive way may channel anger and resentment toward his partner, or toward women in general, resulting in sexual malfunction. This withholding of sexual pleasure can be meant, either consciously or unconsciously, as a form of punishment of the partner. It also guards the man against intimacy. His sexual behavior is really little different from the way he deals with other life events and may represent a general difficulty in dealing with negative feelings appropriately.

Another profile is the narcissistic personality style. A man with this style tends to interact with the world primarily as it reflects his own needs. The world and the people in it are there for his enjoyment. For him, sex can be both a matter of self-satisfaction and a measure of his self-worth. Not only does his sexual performance provide a measure of himself as a man, but his partner's response to him can also be an important indicator of his manhood. To such a man, erectile failure is a significant issue.

POWER, TRUST, AND INTIMACY: WHERE THE PROBLEMS LIE

When relationships develop and deepen, they are usually accompanied by a growing set of expectations. Some of these expectations are common, and are discussed and agreed upon by the partners, while others are unspoken but understood. Examples are agreed-upon understandings about where to live, how to handle finances, how many children to have. Some expectations are privately known only to one partner, but the other is in some way held accountable for these expectations. A woman may think to herself, for example, that her fiancé will cut back on his drinking once they get married. He may expect that she will relax the uptight attitude about sex that she learned from her mother and her church. At a deeper level, some expectations are unknown to either partner and operate at a level outside of conscious awareness. Examples include expecting to be affirmed or rescued by one's partner, or finding that longed-for good-parent figure in one's spouse. These sets of expectations can lead to misunderstanding between partners, especially when it comes to sex. It is here that the three most important elements in a relationship surface: power, trust, and intimacy. The sexual lives of men and women are greatly influenced by these three elements.

Power refers not only to a struggle for control, but also to questions like: Am I respected by my partner? Do I count? Are my feelings and wishes taken into consideration? Is there a balance or sharing in decision making?

Trust refers not only to a degree of comfort about sexual fidelity to the relationship, but also to matters such as financial responsibility, respecting appropriate boundaries of a personal nature, accepting responsibility for chores and parenting issues, being able to "depend" on the other.

Intimacy is the capacity to hear, share, respect, and communicate what is important, whether in sexual matters or life issues in general. It also includes a level of intimacy with oneself, being in touch not only with what one is feeling about sex and one's partner, but also with how those feelings are played out in the relationship. Both popular and scientific literature today speak of gender differences in communication styles. Intimacy skills provide the foundation for many of the issues addressed in power and trust. When men are experiencing erection problems, the psychological causes often reside in the relationship as it plays out the three themes of power, trust, and intimacy.

IS THERE A PURPOSE FOR ERECTILE FAILURE?

Therapists may surprise their patients if they ask them if they see a purpose in their impotence problem. What possible purpose could erectile failure serve except to increase stress and frustration for the man and his partner? When it comes to sex and relationships, it seems that even problems can really represent an adaptation to another problem. In this regard, erectile problems are no different. Think about John, the young man we described at the beginning of this chapter. When he developed potency problems with Carol, what purpose do you think they served in the relationship? Think about it. We will come back to it.

There is an awareness among some sex therapists today, prompted by the observations of Dr. Joseph LoPiccolo, one of the innovators in the field, that focusing just on eliminating presenting symptoms and complaints may be missing the larger picture. The focus on "symptoms" may also be behind many treatment failures. Very often the "couple system" is being kept in balance because of the sexual problem. How can that be? The sexual problem may maintain a balance in the couple because the man's impotence protects both the man and the woman from having to deal with passionate intimacy or the real exploration of their sexual potential. Any underlying conflict about male intimacy with a partner is avoided by having the "symptom." For John and Carol this may have meant that John's erectile problems would keep him from dealing with the possible threat to his sexuality that Carol's sexual responsiveness represented to him. Carol's open enjoyment of sex was a threat to John precisely because it made him face his fears of letting go sexually.

If the female partner is uncomfortable with sex, her partner's impotence allows the couple to covertly avoid dealing with significant sexual and personal issues. From what we said earlier about an individual's sexual development, we can see that there are times when the "cause" of impotence and other male (or female) sexual dysfunctions lies beyond the penis. We will discuss this further in Chapter 15 when we explore the ongoing difficulties that some couples have after the erection problems are "cured."

RELATIONSHIPS: THE PENIS DOESN'T LIE

Most men's sexual lives are played out in their sexual relationships. It is here where they come together, for better or for worse, in intimate contact with a partner. And here lies the problem. All sexual relationships are intimate, whether we are willing to admit it or not. Even casual sex has an intimate component to it, for it involves a sharing of our personal sexual self with another. Both the sexual self and the relationship may or may not be healthy. We can label it "just sex" and maybe even function well, for the "person" is not involved, "just the genitals." Some men do not appreciate the difference. They may "do okay" with a casual partner but have difficulty in an ongoing or committed relationship. For our discussion, let us focus on what happens in a sexual relationship where the man is having erection difficulties with his regular partner.

There are many partner issues that influence sexual performance. Any couple interaction, from verbal expression to nonverbal body language, and all that lies between, can influence how we feel sexually about our partners and ourselves. These feelings can become internalized and influence our sexual interest and sexual response to the partner. This means that over time, unresolved differences can lead to anger and resentment by the spouse. Some men can turn off to such negative emotions and turn on to sexual situations in an automatic way. Other men cannot so easily dismiss negative feelings, and they greatly interfere with their sexual appetite and functioning. Thus nonsexual couple conflict can lead to a decrease in sexual desire, as well as interference with arousal and erection, even when "all the plumbing is working."

If there are no nonsexual complaints about a partner that could be transferred into the sexual relationship, there still might exist a number of areas of sexual concerns or difficulties that, given time, could result in erectile or other dysfunctions. These difficulties often relate to the couple's "sexual script," a term we previously used to describe the way couples view and structure their sexual behavior. Their sexual script determines what sexual behaviors they will engage in and under what circumstances. In fact, a couple's sexual script will have a lot to do with what fosters and maintains desire and arousal. Problems with desire and arousal lead to erectile problems. The penis doesn't lie!

There are a number of sexual difficulties couples can have: partners choosing inconvenient times for sex; inability to relax; disinterest or indifference to sex; disagreement on sexual habits or practices; introducing new lovemaking techniques; use of sexual toys or erotic material or videos in their sexual repertoire; too little or unpleasant foreplay before intercourse; too little tenderness after intercourse; unrealistic expectations of oneself or one's partner; disagreement on frequency of sex. Such disagreements are often at the heart of a couple's problems.

There is no question that men and women are often in both relationship and life-demand "overload." Their sexual life becomes entangled and swept up into the rest of their busy life. In fact it can be said that modern lifestyles conspire against our sex lives. There are times when an attempt at sexual initiation by the male is met with annoyance and dismissal by his partner. At even a modest slight, some men respond with anger and withdraw. Even if the couple does eventually get around to attempting intercourse, he may be so angry that he has difficulty with his erection. Men frequently complain that their partner misinterprets playful affection as a sexual invitation. In this scenario a man may playfully touch, fondle, or say something of a sexual nature to his partner, with no intention of going any further, only to be met with a complaint or accusation—"How could you be thinking about having sex now!" Clearly there has been a misunderstanding here, and if it is not properly addressed, the couple could be on a path that leads to resentment, sexual avoidance, and, ultimately, failure to perform.

Many negative feelings toward the partner are expressed through erectile failure. We keep saying that in many cases the penis doesn't lie! It is hard for a man to get hard when he is angry, frustrated, feeling unappreciated or taken for granted. Women reading this list may well be seeing some of their own issues with their partner. It goes both ways. Men and their partners need to examine the nature of negative feeling that may be behind their sexual complaints. Some issues can be resolved through open and supportive discussion. For example, are other family members interfering with the relationship? If neither partner has separated from family and friends sufficiently that the couple feels "really together," then this should be addressed. Loyalty conflicts between one's partner and one's family and friends can cause more than sexual problems in a relationship. Every couple is different in this regard, but it remains a critical issue for many partners.

Other problems men face that could affect potency involve personal tastes and aesthetics, such as a partner gaining too much weight, or showing the effects of aging. Often their avoidance of sex or poor performance creates personal embarrassment, for they may truly love their partners. Still, they nevertheless find themselves turned off by "something about their partner" and can as a result develop erectile problems. From our brief discussion of couple factors related to erectile failure, it becomes clear that some causes for failure relate directly to a man's feelings about his partner, while others represent a conflict within the man himself.

THE NEW PARTNER SYNDROME

Finding a new sexual partner should be a great thing! Right? Not always. The sexual satisfaction gained in finding a new partner will depend on several factors. First, there are those men who rediscover potency once they have a new partner. They may come back later with a complaint, but not at first. There are other men who, after a brief initial bout of performance anxiety with a new partner, regain their erections at a mutually satisfying level. Good for them. They did not overreact with anxiety, they had a reassuring partner, or both. We should also mention those men who, after an initial failure with a new partner, never go back to see her. This can leave both partners wondering, "Was it me?" In this case, if he carries over the fear of failure to his next sexual encounter, he could be in for trouble. Worry only makes it worse. He may start "watching himself do it," getting more anxious each time, and may end up making sex a spectator sport. But this is obvious. There are more complicated circumstances. He may have found the new partner to be such a "hot number" that he is intimidated by her and doubts his ability to perform. She might be so gorgeous or sexy that he may think she has had many lovers with great and massive erections. She really likes sex, or at least knows great sex when she has it. When a man finds himself filled with these thoughts and doubts, it becomes a sure recipe for erectile failure. As a result, the woman of his dreams may have to remain just one of his fantasies.

Some men who are searching for a new companion are doing so after a painful divorce, relationship breakup, or death of a spouse, leaving them wounded and cautious about intimacy. When these men find a new partner, they often report episodes of erectile failure. Sometimes they have sufficient erections but have difficulty ejaculating, leading to confusion and frustration. At times they have trouble obtaining an initial erection, or they may lose it shortly after entering their partner. These men are not happy about the situation. Sometimes the sexual complaint occurs in a new relationship that otherwise is loving and compatible, and places a cloud over their future together. What is going on?

In a sense, some of these men are still dealing with leftover and unresolved feelings about their previous partner. They may be interrupting their level of arousal with any number of concerns, including anger toward women (their other women); ambivalence about becoming emotionally involved or committed again; feeling unfaithful to the memory of a deceased spouse or partner; discomfort with the level of sexual pleasure they are having; discomfort with the high level of arousal of their new partner, which is beyond what they were used to in their previous partner; and fear of sexual failure and eventual rejection by this new woman. These men need to be told that when it comes to sex, you can't be in two places at once. They are interrupting their own sexual enjoyment and their focus on the present with concerns about the past.

These concerns can be addressed, but it may take time and require patience in both the man and his new partner. Adjusting to a new partner requires a man to examine a number of factors. A man needs to pause to reflect about his opinions about himself as a sexual person, his attitudes toward female sexuality, and his whole sexual script. Part of the required reevaluation will make him question many aspects of sex that he took for granted, especially if the new partner represents a challenge in her open enjoyment of sex. Some changes in attitude and behavior may have to be made. In a sense, he should *hasten slowly*, trust his ability to have erections, and take his time in making the changes in thinking and behavior that will move him toward sexual health. When he has done so, he may be pleasantly surprised with the return of his erectile capacity. His new partner will be pleased—and both will be grateful.

THE SEXUAL SITUATION: TIME, PLACE, AND PERSON

So many men try to have sex under the wrong circumstances and end up frustrated when their erections won't cooperate. This is such a fundamental principle of sexual functioning that one wonders why many men (and women) don't get it! In other words, there is a failure to understand some of the basic principles both of relating to a partner and of how we function as sexual beings. To continue to attempt sex under adverse circumstances is evidence of just how little knowledge many men have about their own sexual functioning. Even if these men have sufficient knowledge, they often do not use common sense in applying it to their sex lives. Remember, sexual capacity is subject to the same forces of physiology and circumstance as the rest of our functioning. Attempting sex when one is too tired, too rushed, too angry, too annoyed, too bored, too preoccupied, too ambivalent, too guilty, not really sufficiently interested or aroused, after too much to drink or eat, without proper privacy, in the wrong surroundings, and even with the wrong partner is inviting situational erectile failure.

There are probably other circumstances that apply as well, but there is no doubt that men set themselves up for failure when they engage in sex under adverse circumstances. This situational failure should not be a cause for alarm. Learn from it. While it may be a missed opportunity for sexual pleasure, it is not the end of one's sex life.

While most men would probably understand why an adverse circumstance—such as drinking too much—would cause erectile failure, they do not usually understand how routine aspects of their lifestyle can also be contributors to failure. Many men develop erectile problems because they fail to recognize that their lifestyle conspires against their sex lives. For many couples, whether they have children or not, sex usually comes at the end of a busy day, after the eleven-o'clock news, when both partners are tired, or even exhausted. Even if the man is able to have an erection, he may not be sufficiently aroused to sustain it. Men should know that having an erection does not mean that they are sufficiently aroused to attempt intercourse. The older a man gets, the more truth he will see in this statement.

A good example that the presence of an erection does not always equal arousal is the normal occurrence of nocturnal and morning erections. The erection may be adequate, but the desire and arousal for sex, if it happens at all, comes later, depending on the circumstances. The best therapeutic intervention for men who are faced with a busy lifestyle is to advise them to be realistic about sex and to plan or look for opportunities when their time together with their partner will support their being sexual. More about this in Chapter 12.

Many men think they should be ready to have sex at any time. Sex therapist Bernie Zilbergeld refers to this as the male fantasy model of sex. The truth, of course, is that not all men are always ready for sex. This truth becomes especially clear when men attempt intercourse with the wrong partner. The choice of a sexual partner, either in a casual meeting with a new person or in a chance encounter with someone already known, does not always lead to a satisfactory time together.

Factors such as anxiety, guilt, or certain personal insecurities can quickly short-circuit the male sexual response.

There are also phases of life or developmental markers that can influence a man's capacity for erection. A partial list of these markers include coping with sex during pregnancy or a partner's illness; a change in the relationship because of the birth of a child or, later, when the children leave home; adjusting to a new job, the loss of a job, or home relocation; divorce or relationship separation or termination; and death of a spouse or significant family member. Many of these developmental events are an unavoidable part of life, and they can contribute to a decrease of sexual desire or reduced erectile functioning.

Men can also experience erectile failure with someone who is an inappropriate partner choice because of any number of factors, including age, sex, religious differences, race, body type, reputation, even career or socioeconomic status. Whatever the cause, the resulting erectile failure can cause men unnecessary concern. If they are able to distance themselves and their "male ego" from the situation, they will see that the difficulty lay in their partner choice, not in their overall ability to have adequate erections. Some men are even able to see some humor in the experience. Having a sense of humor about sex can go a long way toward keeping oneself sexually healthy and happy.

The psychological causes and resulting effects of impotence are varied and at times very complicated. The overview we have presented can help men focus with more clarity on what causes their own unique difficulty. Once this is understood, men can begin to get back on the road to sexual health.

6

PHYSICAL CAUSES OF IMPOTENCE

I am still learning.
—*Michelangelo*

Key Points:

Most cases of impotence are due to a combination of physical and psychological factors.

The most common physical causes of impotence are:

1. Vascular conditions
2. Alcohol
3. Medications
4. Diabetes
5. Abnormal nerve function
6. Hormone deficiency
7. Removal of the prostate gland for cancer
8. Other surgical procedures
9. Peyronie's disease
10. Illicit drugs
11. Smoking and diet, as contributing factors

It is not always possible to make a clear distinction between psychological and physical causes. Even cases in which there is an obvious physical cause for the problem, psychological issues are often found, but only if one delves into the matter.

Traditionally, it has been considered important to separate physical and psychological causes of impotence as well as to separate treatment recommendations according to the cause. Patients whose impotence was felt to have psychological causes were generally advised to have counseling or sex therapy. Patients whose impotence was due to physical causes initially had only a penile prosthesis and later a vacuum constriction device to consider as treatment options. Although newer forms of therapy have evolved that are suitable for treating impotence regardless of whether it is psychological or physical, this book, for ease of understanding, makes the traditional separation into "physical" and "psychological" for both causes and treatment.

VASCULAR CAUSES

> The sky is not less blue because a blind man does
> not see it.
>
> —*Author unknown*

Unlike the whale, walrus, and dog, which have a bone in the penis, human males rely on the inflow of blood to create expansion and rigidity. Any process that impairs the inflow of blood can cause impotence. Examples are hardening of the arteries (atherosclerosis), diabetes, and high blood pressure. A less common cause is Peyronie's disease, in which scar tissue forms in the erectile compartments of the penis.

Since a successful erection depends upon storage of blood to cause distention of the erectile tissue in the penis, leakage of blood may also cause impotence. Individuals who have "venous leakage" may have no trouble getting blood into the penis but do have a problem storing it. In short, the blood that enters the erectile tissue of the penis empties too quickly into veins, preventing an erection. These two vascular problems—poor blood inflow and too rapid blood outflow—are the most common causes of impotence.

As research progresses, it is apparent that the erectile mechanism is more complex than previously thought. In some cases, abnormalities in the internal structure of the penis may prevent an erection. For example, the smooth muscle of blood vessels, normally in a constricted state, may not be able to relax and allow blood to enter the penis, or the outside lining of the erectile compartments (tunica albuginea) may become scarred and not function properly. Even the erectile tissue itself, which may be thought of as spongelike, may become damaged and not accept or store blood properly. As scientists continue to unravel the mechanisms of erection dysfunction, more and more treatment options will become available.

ALCOHOL

Lechery Sir, it provokes and unprovokes;
it provokes the desire but takes away performance.
—*Shakespeare*

The above comment about alcohol, made by the porter in *Macbeth* (Act II, Scene III), tells us that even in Shakespeare's time it was clear what effect alcohol has upon erections. That alcohol is an impediment to erections comes as a surprise to many men. Some males rely upon alcohol to "loosen them up" and make them more outgoing. Then, to their disappointment, they find they cannot perform sexually. What they don't understand is that alcohol is a depressant, not a stimulant, to the central nervous system. The chronic use of alcohol may exert adverse effects by causing nerve damage, liver failure through cirrhosis, and a generalized state of malnutrition, all of which may contribute to impotence. In addition, the testicles may shrink and cease to function properly. As one alcoholic said, "I started out like Early Times but ended up like Old Granddad."

Alcohol should not be ingested in significant quantities if a male has had any difficulties achieving erections. However, in limited amounts, it is not harmful. No precise guidelines can be provided as to the quantities of alcohol one can ingest, because, like sex, what is too much for one man isn't enough for another. Unfortunately, as a man becomes intoxicated, there are no warning signals to tell him that he has reached the point at which he will be unable to perform sexually. Some men learn from experience; others do not.

IS THE CAUSE OF YOUR IMPOTENCE IN YOUR MEDICINE CABINET?

Leave the life there in its ease, let it take care of itself, it will do better than if you paralyze it by loading it with medicine.

—*Napoleon*

There is a great deal of medication use in our society. Some of our most important and commonly used drugs can have adverse side effects, including impotence. Some of these medicines may also delay or stop ejaculation altogether. Others may cause a decrease in libido.

If you have a problem with potency or changes in ejaculation or sex drive (libido), your medications should be reviewed with your physician. Drugs of many classes have been associated with erection difficulties: antidepressants, blood pressure medications, drugs for peptic ulcer, hormones, sedatives, anti-anxiety agents, narcotics, stimulants, major and minor tranquilizers, estrogens, and even some medications available over the counter for colds and allergies.

While it is reasonable to take the approach that any medication might be the cause of impotence, it is not practical to list every medicine that might be a cause. There are three reasons for this. First is the simple fact that there are many thousands of medicines available that could be a factor, and any attempt to make a comprehensive list would fail. Second, even those medicines that have been known to cause impotence in certain individuals do not affect all men in the same way. Third, if he finds a medicine he takes on a list of medicines that may be associated with impotence, a male struggling to find the cause of his problem might jump to the conclusion that the medicine is the root of his problem, and he may avoid a proper evaluation that could uncover the real cause, or worse, he might stop taking a medication that he truly needs.

The single most important question is this: "Did your sexual problem begin soon after taking a medication?" If the answer is yes, then a properly trained individual must review the particular side effects of that medication. In addition, an attempt must be made to determine if the relationship between the onset of impotence and erectile insufficiency is causal or simply coincidental. Some medicines may affect one man's ability to have an erection but not another's. Hence, each medicine must be considered on an individual basis and each person's response may be considered unique.

If a man is impotent or is having other sexual difficulties, such as decreased libido or inability to ejaculate, then it is important that he discuss his medication with his physician. No patient should discontinue medication without first consulting his physician.

THE EFFECT OF DIABETES ON ERECTIONS

> Life is not a spectacle or a feast;
> it is a predicament.
> —*George Santayana*

Diabetes mellitus is so common in the United States that it deserves special mention. Approximately 50 percent of diabetics will become impotent.

Diabetes interferes with both the neurological and vascular systems to cause erectile insufficiency. The characteristics of impotence in diabetes include the following:

1. The impotence may occur at any age but is most commonly seen between the ages of thirty-five and fifty.
2. It is usually seen in patients who are on insulin but can also be seen in patients using oral agents.
3. The diabetes is usually of relatively long standing—more than ten years.
4. The symptoms of impotence begin slowly and gradually.
5. The symptoms are progressive and become persistent.
6. There is an absence of morning erections.

7. Sex drive is not directly affected.
8. The level of the hormone testosterone is normal.
9. Prior to the onset of impotence, patients may have noted an inability to ejaculate.

PROBLEMS WITH NERVE FUNCTION

> Illness arrives on horseback;
> it departs on foot.
> —*Author Unknown*

There are many factors that can impair the normal transmission of nerve impulses necessary to create an erection. Such problems are seen in patients with diabetes, stroke, spinal cord injury, or diseases of the nervous system such as multiple sclerosis. These factors are complex and may vary among individual patients. A discussion with your doctor will determine whether or not consultation with a physician who specializes in diseases of the nerves, a neurologist, is necessary.

HORMONAL DEFICIENCY

> Life is a gamble with terrible odds.
> If it was a bet, you wouldn't take it.
> —*Tom Stoppard*

Low levels of testosterone in the bloodstream may cause erectile dysfunction—usually a loss of libido. An insufficient level of testosterone is seen in a male whose brain fails to properly stimulate the testicles to produce testosterone or in a male whose testicles are unable to manufacture the hormone. Unless the hormonal level is very low, decreased testosterone is not usually the cause of impotence.

Besides testosterone, other hormones may have an effect on erectile ability. In men with cirrhosis of the liver, there may be high circulating levels of the female hormone estrogen. Many of these men are impotent. A few patients will have a tumor in the pituitary gland, which secretes a hormone called prolactin. This is easily determined with a blood test. Patients who are severely hypothyroid may also complain of impotence. Both conditions are treatable.

REMOVAL OF THE PROSTATE GLAND FOR CANCER

It's not as bad as it sounds.
—*Mark Twain, commenting on Wagner's music*

Patients who undergo treatment for prostate cancer are at risk for the development of impotence. This is true not just for patients who have surgery to remove the prostate but also for those who receive radiation externally or from the implantation of radioactive seeds into the prostate. However, as will be discussed more thoroughly in Chapter 38, it may be necessary to accept erectile problems as a trade-off for a cure from cancer.

Males with prostate cancer that has spread are not generally candidates for radical surgery to remove the prostate gland or radiation treatments in order to effect a cure. If these patients have evidence of spread of the cancer (metastases), they may receive hormonal treatment to lower testosterone levels, since testosterone can fuel the tumor. This can be accomplished by periodic injections or by surgical castration. It should be remembered, however, that low levels of testosterone are generally associated with the loss of sex drive (libido). Impotence may or may not be associated with loss of the testicles in adult life.

Whether patients undergo surgery or radiation to cure prostate cancer, most will find that they are unable to ejaculate. Some men, however, continue to describe the pleasurable feeling of orgasm.

OTHER SURGICAL PROCEDURES

I believe that the only disability in life is a bad
attitude.
—*Scott Hamilton*

Other surgical procedures may cause impotence, particularly if the operation is performed in the pelvis. Examples are removal of the bladder for malignancy and removal of a portion of the lower colon for cancer of the bowel. Surgery on the major blood vessels supplying the legs may also result in loss of potency, since the blood and/or nerve supply to the penis may be interrupted.

PEYRONIE'S DISEASE

The pessimist complains about the wind;
The optimist expects it to change;
The realist adjusts the sails.

—*William Arthur Ward*

Peyronie's disease refers to a condition in which there is dense scar tissue, usually located along the top of the penis, in the erectile cylinders. This condition is named after François de la Peyronie, the physician who first described it in 1743. Curiously, when the penis is soft it appears normal; however, if one feels along the top of the phallus, there is a firm area where the scar is located. This scar causes the penis to angulate when it is erect. In addition to causing curvature, this may cause significant discomfort to the male. If the bend is severe, it may also cause discomfort to the female, since, in effect, during intercourse a curved object rather than a straight one is being thrust into the vagina. The scar may become so rigid and cause such angulation that the male cannot achieve penetration. In mild cases, there is no interference with erections. In more severe cases, patients may develop difficulty attaining and/or sustaining an erection.

Most scarring involves the top part of the erectile compartment of the penis, which causes an upward angulation. If the scar is in fact on the undersurface of the penis, then a downward angulation will result. Lateral bending of the penis occurs when the scar formation is located primarily on one side or the other of the penis. It is not uncommon for patients to complain that the penis does not become rigid between the location of the scar and the head of the penis.

The condition, while not common in the overall population, is most often seen in men in their forties and fifties. Pain is frequently present. However, the discomfort usually disappears within months or years. The degree of penile bend may remain stable, increase, or decrease.

The cause of Peyronie's disease is unknown. However, one theory is that the scar forms as a result of inflammation or injury to the penis. One possible scenario is that a couple frequently engage in intercourse with the female in the superior position. As she lowers her body during thrusting, the rigid penis may be bent so that excess strain is placed upon the erectile tissue. Other experts believe that the impotence associated with Peyronie's disease is due to a defect in the "venous occlusive" mechanism. (See Chapter 4.) Simply stated, the blood that flows into the penis is not trapped in the erection compartment to create distention and rigidity.

It should be emphasized that not every patient with Peyronie's disease will develop impotence. In most patients, the scarring does not progress to the point where vaginal penetration is impossible.

Despite the fact that the condition has been known for more than 250 years, treatment is far from ideal. There is no single approach that gives guaranteed results. Multiple forms of therapy have been tried, including ultrasound, radiation, oral medications, steroid injections, and surgery. Many experts still recommend increased doses of Vitamin E in a dose of 200–400 mg two times a day. The ultimate outcome is unpredictable. Some cases of Peyronie's disease will disappear on their own, and more extreme cases require surgical intervention. This surgery is technically challenging and should be performed only by a highly experienced surgeon.

ILLICIT DRUGS

> The wise learn by others' mistakes;
> fools by their own.
>
> —*Author unknown*

The idea that drugs may enhance sexual pleasure and performance is not a new one. Roman orgies have been well documented in both literature and art. At such orgies, drugs were freely used, and social and sexual inhibitions vanished. But do any illegal drugs really facilitate sexual performance?

Reliable data are hard to come by, because few scientific studies have been conducted. However, we do know certain things about the effects of some commonly used illicit drugs on sexual behavior.

Marijuana

Marijuana, obtained from the flowering tops of hemp plants, has been in use for centuries. Many people claim that their sexual experience is heightened and their performance improved if they smoke marijuana prior to intercourse. This drug does induce a dreamy state in which inhibitions may diminish. Perception is changed, and hallucinations may occur. However, its only apparent role in sex may be that in small doses it reduces anxiety, which may otherwise prevent a male from obtaining an erection.

The negative effects of marijuana have been recognized for a long time. The Indian Hemp Drug Commission of 1894 reported that hemp drugs have "no aphrodisiac power whatsoever and, as a matter of fact, they are used by ascetics in this country with the ostensible objective of destroying sexual appetite." The drug does cause a heightened self-awareness of both thoughts and feelings, which may lead to a disinterest in a relationship with a female partner. Therefore, despite the positive effects claimed by some users, marijuana is not a cure for impotence.

Heroin

Narcotics in general have a harmful effect on sexual performance. Most drug addicts experience impotence, and many others are unable to ejaculate. When the male is "high," he cannot perform sexually. When he is not high, his basic concern—indeed, his obsession—is where he will get his next fix.

The initial sensation following intravenous injection of heroin is pleasure and warmth. An erection may occur, but it usually disappears rapidly. Some men experience such total euphoria that they describe their high as being just like an orgasm. This may replace the need for those feelings that sexual intercourse would provide. Many addicts who can still achieve an erection report that their frequency of sexual intercourse is less than once a month.

Amphetamines

There is evidence that amphetamine use may increase sexual activity. Interestingly, when a male is high on amphetamines, he has little interest in sex. It is only during the withdrawal, or "crashing," that sexual interest or performance is heightened.

Some males report spontaneous erections after an injection of an amphetamine, and many individuals under the influence of amphetamines describe their sexual experience as being prolonged. Many report an increase in libido as well. However, these drugs are not without harmful side effects. Confusion, hallucinations, panic states, homicidal tendencies, and fatal convulsions may occur. The drugs should be considered dangerous and avoided.

LSD

LSD is not noted for enhancing sexual performance. It may cause sexual hallucinations, but performance is generally more difficult because the user cannot concentrate on reality long enough to accomplish anything. For every individual who feels that his sexual experience is enhanced, there is another who feels that LSD has detracted from his sexual performance.

Cocaine

Hard-core users of cocaine usually develop sexual difficulties, and impotence is not uncommon. Cocaine produces an anesthetic effect and has been used by some males as an aid to prolonging intercourse before ejaculation. It is rubbed on the head of the penis just prior to insertion and may permit more vigorous thrusting before a male ejaculates. However, it may be harmful to the female and it does not help with erections.

SMOKING AND DIET

> The progress of rivers to the sea is not as rapid as
> that of man to error.
>
> *—Voltaire*

There is no longer any question about the harmful effects of smoking on male sexual function. Damage to the arteries carrying blood to the penis may occur. Exposure to cigarette smoking, either first hand or possibly second hand, is associated with progression of atherosclerosis, and the impact is greater in men who already have diabetes or high blood pressure.

The same dietary excesses that damage blood vessels to the heart will harm the penis, namely a diet high in fat and cholesterol. Thus smoking and a high-fat diet have a common denominator in causing impotence. Both damage blood vessels, which results in a reduction of blood flow to the erectile bodies of the penis.

7

MYTHS AND FALLACIES THAT PROMOTE IMPOTENCE

I would rather have my ignorance than another man's knowledge because I have got so much more of it.
—*Mark Twain*

Key Points:

- Myths about sex are based on ignorance and misinformation. Males learn early in their lives that performance counts.
- There are many myths that men have about sex, including: men are always ready for sex; foreplay must lead to sex, erections should be automatic; men are responsible for what goes on during sex and real sex requires having good erections.
- Other myths: masturbation causes impotence; penile length is a measure of masculinity; during intercourse the penis can be locked in the vagina; vasectomy causes impotence.

Where do our myths about sexuality come from? Many are rooted in gender stereotypes and cultural expectations. Some come through the media. No matter the source, faulty attitudes and sexual ignorance based on sexual misinformation can lead to erectile dysfunction. Sexual attitudes are learned. What we learn can very easily become part of our "automatic" feelings and are lived out in our behavior. Unfortunately, many men (and women) are trying to live out their sexual lives while being guided by a faulty and out-of-date road map. They may be lost and not even know it! After a while, there is little attempt to refute or correct the inaccurate beliefs. In part, this is because myths deal with what can be very personal to us and speak to us at a very deep level: the level of personal validation.

We easily buy into what the myths say to us because they hold up a standard to achieve. We will know whether we are good enough. But by whose rules? Who says so? The myths? In other words, it is very easy to embrace unquestioningly a popular myth about sex as a goal to be attained. After all, men (and women) like goals. They tell us where we stand when compared to others. Everyone loves a winner—especially when it comes to sexual performance and success. But embracing the unrealistic expectation of sexual myths can set us up to feel like losers.

While we may understand where the roots of sexual myths come from, there is no question that they are based on an astonishing amount of misinformation. Until fairly recently, it was difficult to gain access to detailed information about sexual functioning. Not until sex education classes became the norm was this information readily available. As a result, the sexual education of most men over fifty was picked up in the schoolyard or from pornographic magazines and films. Sex education classes simply did not exist for them. This lack of knowledge is one of the major factors contributing to erectile insufficiency. Many men were given grossly erroneous information, and they tended to pass it along. Art Buchwald has satirized this situation well:

> I had no formal sex education when I was a student. . . . We got all our sex education at the local candy store after 3:00. The information was dispensed by 13 year olds who seemed to know everything there was to know on the subject, and we 11 and 12 year olds believed every word they told us. . . . For example. . . the method of kissing a girl on the mouth determined whether she would become pregnant or not. Every time I kissed a girl after that I sweated for the next nine months. . . . When I turned 13, I became an instructor myself and passed on my knowledge to 11 and

12 year olds at the same candy store....I was amazed with how much authority I was able to pass on the facts of life as I knew them....We were all emotional wrecks before we got to high school.

THE FANTASY MODEL OF SEX

Sigmund Freud is often quoted as saying that a woman's anatomy is her destiny. Cannot this statement also apply to men? In an earlier chapter, we spoke about gender roles and expectations, and how from a very early age, boys are socialized to perform and perform well. In other words, performance counts.

Traditionally, boys have been raised with the message that they should avoid being weak, dependent, or demonstrative of tender feelings. Certainly, contemporary thinking is beginning to put these notions to rest. Nevertheless, boys are often led to believe that they should be able to do anything, and this sense of expected omnipotence can lead to farfetched myths about sexual prowess. The Catch-22 is that these myths, rather than leading to peak performance, can prevent a man from functioning well sexually. Therefore, eliminating sexual myths and fallacies is essential to allow a man the sense of freedom to "be himself" in his sexual relationships instead of trying to live up to an unrealistic sexual standard.

The overall myth that affects sexual performance is called the "fantasy model of sex." It provides a road map that is nearly impossible to follow. It is centered on male sexual performance, and the performance itself is centered around the notion of a large, automatically functioning penis. The bigger the better, and use it to knock her socks off! The penis has a job to do. You need the right equipment to do it. That means a man's penis is fully functional, and ready whenever and wherever it is needed.

This is a daunting expectation for most men to have of themselves. This model implies that sex isn't for enjoyment, or expressing love and caring. Sex becomes a way for proving oneself as a man. A performance model like this stresses that penis size, hardness, and endurance and frequent orgasms are all necessary to enthrall the partner. Rather than considering sex as an expression of feelings and enjoyment, this model focuses on doing. Even if many men do not fully accept this stereotypic myth, it may still be on their minds whenever they do not "measure up" to the task. Erectile failures quickly become a devastating blow to self-esteem.

Let us explore some of the more common sexual myths. These myths tend to cluster in the beliefs about penile size, performance, functioning, aging, quality of sex, and role and function of women.

Myth: Men are always ready for sex.

This belief can lead to tremendous unhappiness. Men do not have to always be ready, or interested, in sex, even when the opportunity presents itself. The truth is that men are subject to swings in the degree of their desire and interest in sex. Fatigue, partner issues, business concerns, and distractions all may influence a man's interest and readiness for sex. A man should be honest with himself. Most men are not horny all the time. This is especially true as men age. A man is being unfair to himself and his partner if he attempts intercourse when he is not ready or in the mood. Doing so can easily lead to a cycle of erectile failure.

Myth: Pleasurable contact must lead to sex.

This expectation causes many problems for men and their partners. Not that the urge to keep going is not there, but it may be enough for the partner just to engage in pleasurable touching. When men realize this, they will be more willing to engage in extended "outercourse" as a way of sharing pleasure. This "new" attitude will allow them opportunities for closeness when they are not in the mood for intercourse. Men will often find their partners very receptive to this kind of intimacy, since many women find it appealing. In fact, it is not uncommon for women to complain that while they enjoy closeness and pleasurable touching, they often avoid contact with their partner because "he always wants to go all the way." Touching and being touched are a wonderful part of being human, and need not always be a prelude to sex. Men should be careful not to place this expectation on themselves or their partner.

Myth: Real sex requires that a man have a good erection.

Many men will stop sexual activity if they feel they have not become hard enough for penetration. It is as if all the pleasure of foreplay did not count because there may not be a "main event." This interruption of sexual activity can reinforce anxiety about getting an erection the next time. On the other hand, it is reasonable not to attempt intercourse if one is not sufficiently aroused. The point here is that there are many ways of mutual pleasure that do not require an erection. Mutual pleasure builds closeness and trust. Such intimate closeness can be tremendously satisfactory, which is one of the benefits of a sexual experience—for both partners.

Myth: Erections should be automatic.

Wrong again. Despite the performance expectations that are central to so many steamy novels, adult videos, and early memories of puberty, erections are not always automatic. This is especially true in long-term relationships and as an accompaniment of aging. It is true that a new partner and novel situations might provide the extra psychic stimulation to give many men an erection boost. Yet, the reality is that men may require direct stimulation to the penis by their partner in order to obtain an erection. Failure to understand this may lead to real erection problems because men can wonder "what is wrong with me" when they do not get an erection on their own. This can lead to excessive worry about the next sexual encounter, and that worry, of course, can lead to erectile failure.

Myth: If a man has an erection, he is ready for sex.

Not true. The most common nonsexual erection occurs in the middle of the night or in the early morning. These erections are part of a nightly sleeping pattern (during REM sleep) and are nature's way of keeping the erectile tissue healthy by supplying oxygen-rich blood to the penis. Having this type of erection does not always mean that the man is psychically aroused enough to have intercourse. He may not be fully roused emotionally. And he may or may not become further aroused once he realizes that he has an erection. If he acts too quickly, without sufficient attention to both his arousal and his partner, he may lose his erection. If erection loss happens, then "he woke her up for nothing." Where that would lead depends on the state of the relationship of the couple.

Myth: Sex should lead to orgasm.

Many men feel that once sexual activity has been initiated, orgasm must follow—certainly for him, preferably for her too, and why not simultaneously? This myth fails to take into account that a sexual experience can be satisfying without orgasm. Women know this. Men have trouble understanding what a woman means when she says that the closeness of the union was satisfying, and that not having an orgasm was okay. Younger men in particular have difficulty with this notion because they tend to be orgasm-focused and refuse to believe a partner's insistence that no orgasm was necessary. For men of all ages, needing to constantly go all the way to orgasm eliminates variety in lovemaking, including taking a break to rest and talk, or to restimulate each other to higher levels of arousal.

What men also do not tend to appreciate is that as they age, the urge to ejaculate during sex is not as strong as it was when they were younger. Thus their lovemaking and sexual script have to be expanded to include intercourse that allows for a satisfying closeness but may not always lead to orgasm. Remember, for partners who have regular access to each other, there is always tomorrow. Do not panic. Enjoy the pleasure of the present situation. Once couples appreciate this, they may discover the comfort and intimacy of brief interludes of vaginal penetration without the demand to continue to orgasm. For some men, this practice provides a nice way to begin or end the day with their partners. As for simultaneous orgasm, making it a goal can be risky, especially when one considers how many women can "normally" have difficulty having an orgasm during intercourse. To deal with this, many couples develop their own comfort level with who comes first, at all, or together. The key point here is that explosive simultaneous orgasms may certainly occur, but satisfying sexual encounters can be achieved without them.

Myth: Sexual performance should come naturally and be spontaneous.

Experience should tell men that thinking this way can result in frustration and failure. Like it or not, men can *learn* how to be better lovers, not only in terms of technique, but also in understanding themselves and their partners as sexual persons. Both men and women say that the spontaneity of sex is romantic and to plan it takes much of the romance away. But the reality is that planning a sexual activity can also add special dimension to lovemaking by heightening the anticipation. Planning also helps busy partners avoid the failure and disappointment of trying to be "spontaneously" sexual rather than waiting until they truly want to have sex. It often pays to admit that the best time for sex is when rested on a weekend and when time to be together can be planned and unhurried. As a way of anticipation, other time spent together can focus on keeping the erotic pot bubbling with words, touches, and other intimate ways of showing and building desire.

Myth: Men are responsible for what goes on during sex.

Belief in this myth places a burden on the man at the same time it negates the woman's right to be sexual. The corollary to this myth is that women should be passive and please their partners, even at the expense of their own pleasure. Today's woman speaks up much more forcefully than her counterpart in the past, but many men are still not listening and are taking on much more responsibility for what happens during sex than is necessary. Sex is a shared responsibility.

Myth: If you love your partner, sex will not become boring.

This myth presents a real double bind for both partners. A man's functioning and ability to become aroused will be seriously affected if he feels his sex life is monotonous. The truth is that even very loving couples can get into a dull routine in their lovemaking. That's because relationships often become predictable. Predictability can lead to boredom, and boredom can result in erectile failure. Men in these circumstances tend to rationalize their situation by saying they are "just getting old," or they may look elsewhere for a little passion.

When it comes to looking outside of the relationship, they usually find out one of two things: extrarelational sex is exciting, which should not be a surprise; or the sex with a new partner only made them feel guilty and more confused, which should also not be a surprise. If they experienced an anxiety-induced bout of impotence during their extracurricular sexual activity, these men then have to deal with the new fear of "what is really wrong with me?" They may end up with

more problems than when they started. The presence of sexual boredom in a long-term relationship is to be expected. The monotony
should not be used as an excuse to withdraw further from sex. Men
need to be reminded that sex is never simple, and they should talk the
problem over with their partner. Their sexual script may need review-
ing to see where some of the problem areas lie. In an otherwise good
relationship, the effort is worth it.

Myth: Masturbation causes baldness, warts, insanity, and impotence.

Masturbation has been condemned throughout the ages. Some
believe that this proscription has its roots in the Bible. The Book of
Genesis relates that Onan utilized withdrawal as a means of contraception. This wasteful "spilling of the seed" infuriated God, who therefore
struck Onan dead. While Onan's real sin was not masturbation but
coitus interruptus, the term "onanism" has become synonymous with
"masturbation."

During the eighteenth century, masturbation was thought to cause
insanity and fatal illness. Masturbation was so ill regarded that some
men who could not desist actually committed suicide. At that time, it
was believed that prevention was the only way to avoid the torments
that were certain to follow masturbation. Some physicians of the day
advocated cutting the nerves that lead to the penis in order to prevent
erections. The fact that the male would then be impotent was acceptable, since it meant that he had been spared far greater distress. In
Europe, between 1800 and 1850, many instruments were designed to
prevent masturbation. Some were constructed of metal and leather and
covered the genitalia so securely that a male could not touch his penis.
Others took the form of spike-like rings that fit so snugly over the penis
that if an erection occurred, the spikes would dig into the skin. These
rings could even be worn at night, so that if an erection occurred while
the male was asleep, he would be suddenly awakened. Another device
consisted of a metal cage that fit over the penis and permitted erections, but had closely fitting bars, so that it was difficult to grasp the
phallus and masturbate. However, as an extra precaution, this device
was sold with handcuffs. In the early part of the twentieth century, a

nurse invented one of the most surefire devices of all. The male was fitted into a leather jacket and pants. The pants were lined with steel armor. Urine escaped through perforated holes in the metal, but a separate trapdoor in the rear, which was padlocked, had to be released by another individual to permit defecation.

In France, in the 1750s, S. A. Tissot cited masturbation as a cause of impotence. In addition, he suggested that masturbation resulted in other serious complications such as loss of vision, indigestion, and mental illness. Dr. Benjamin Rush, a nationally prominent physician of his time, suggested in 1830 that a great sexual appetite would produce impotence. He stated: "When indulged in, an undue or promiscuous intercourse will produce sexual weakness, impotence . . . and death." H. Boerhaave, a Dutch physician who practiced in the early eighteenth century, warned that "the semen discharged too lavishly occasions a weariness, a weakness, an indisposition of motion, convulsions, dryness, pains in the membrane of the brain, dullness of the senses, tabes dorsalis [syphilis], foolishness, and impotence." The *Boy Scout Manual* of 1945 advised boys to "avoid wasting the vital fluid."

At some time or other, masturbation has been blamed for nearly all of the world's evils. Men have been taught to expect baldness, warts on their hands, and blindness if they masturbate. It is therefore no surprise that impotence has also been attributed to masturbation.

Despite all the myths and old wives' tales, it can be firmly stated that masturbation does not cause impotence. In some cases, if a man derives more pleasure from masturbation than from intercourse, it may affect his interest in available sexual relationships and become his primary means of sexual gratification. However, it does not affect his ability to have an erection.

Myth: Masturbation ends with marriage. If you need to do it, there is something wrong.

This myth is a variation on the adolescent boast, "I don't have to jerk off, I can get laid." Masturbation and intercourse are not mutually exclusive. It is common for men to feel guilty if they masturbate and they keep it a secret from their wives or partners. If the partner discovers the behavior, she may take this normal behavior as a sign that she is not sexually satisfying her partner. In some cases this is true, especially, of course, if she often refuses sex and the man prefers masturbation to infidelity.

In most cases, however, masturbation simply provides an opportunity to be sexual, or to relieve sexual tension. Masturbation also provides a man with the confidence of knowing that his erectile response is intact. Some studies suggest that frequent ejaculation also encourages a man's body to stimulate its testosterone level. Sex therapists often recommend masturbation exercises for men in the treatment of impotence and premature ejaculation. Life experience tells us that both partners may not always want to be sexual at the same time. The normal practice of masturbation can be part of one's sexuality that is on a continuum—a continuum that also includes sexual intimacy with one's partner.

Masturbation both before marriage and during married life is, in fact, extremely common. In one survey, 90 percent of all males interviewed indicated that they had masturbated at some time in their lives. The highest frequency of masturbation occurred in the group between twenty-five and thirty-four years of age.

Among married men, the report of masturbation has increased since Kinsey's data of the 1940s. Kinsey showed that more than 40 percent of married men between the ages of twenty-six and thirty-five masturbated, with a median frequency of six times a year. In the 1970s more than 70 percent of all married men masturbated, with a median frequency of twenty-four times a year.

Men and women are sexual beings whether or not they have a partner. In fact, some sex therapists encourage partners to masturbate with and in front of each other as part of their sexual script. This practice provides the couple with alternatives to intercourse while teaching each what pleases the other. Many women today find that masturbation is a valuable asset in learning about their bodies and what variety of sexual stimulation pleases them. These private sexual practices, often including the use of a vibrator, can assist women in discovering and enhancing their orgasmic response. Women can bring these newly learned skills to be mutually enjoyed and shared with their partner.

Myth: Penile length is a measure of masculinity.

This is a myth that causes a great deal of concern among men. Nearly every man has wondered, at some point, whether his penis is too short. Some men shy away from sexual intercourse because they feel that their phallus is of insufficient length to satisfy their partner or they worry that they will be found inadequate in comparison with other males.

Curiosity about penis size is well documented. In 1935, Oliva Dionne, who had fathered quintuplets, was followed into the bathroom at the Congress Hotel in Chicago by curious onlookers who hoped to get a view of what was alleged to be an extraordinarily large phallus. Jokes about Papa Dionne were widespread:

> *While visiting a fair Papa Dionne asked to see a prized bull which was very well endowed. "Listen" he was told, "it's no problem. The bull just asked to see you."*

In our society, men treat penises like income: You don't ask a man how much money he makes or how long his penis is. But while a man will rarely discuss whether his penis is long or short, few will hesitate to tell a good joke about the subject:

> *Attractive woman: "I am not going to bed with any man unless he has twelve inches!"*
> *Propositioning male: "Sorry, but I am not cutting off four inches for any woman."*

It is widely thought by both men and women that penile length varies tremendously. It doesn't. Scientific studies have shown that in the nonerect state, the normal penis measures between approximately three and one-third inches to just over four inches, with an average of almost three and three-quarters inches. The average erect penis is six inches long, although it varies from four and a half to eight inches.

It is also commonly believed that a penis that is large in its flaccid state will show a proportionally greater increase in length when erect than a smaller penis. In fact, the opposite is true. Shorter penises may show a slightly greater proportional increase in length than longer ones.

Another erroneous belief is that big penises belong only to physically big men. However, skeletal and muscular development do not necessarily correlate with penile length. In one scientific study the largest penis was approximately five and a half inches long in the nonerect state even though the patient was only five feet seven inches tall and weighed 152 pounds. And contrary to popular opinion, shoe size is not a reliable predictor for penile length.

It is not uncommon for a urologist to hear a patient express the feeling that he is "underendowed," and for good reason. When a man looks at his own penis it appears smaller than when it is viewed by someone else, simply because of the angle of viewing. A caution to men who have gained weight and increased lower abdominal girth: The penis will *appear* to be shorter. Lose weight and the penis seems to grow.

And does it really matter? Do women really derive greater pleasure during intercourse from a man who has a longer penis? And is a large penis necessarily sexually attractive to a female? There is no doubt that some women may associate a large penis with increased masculinity. But from a strictly physiological standpoint, a longer penis does not necessarily provide more pleasure, because the most sensitive spot for stimulation is near the opening of the vagina. The area farther inside the vagina has very little sensation. Hence, a rather short penis may be just as stimulating in the critical area as a supersized one. And it should not be forgotten that the circumference of the penis may be more important in determining sexual satisfaction for the female than the length, since a larger diameter may have more effect on the female's sensitive areas.

Myth: The penis can become locked in the vagina during intercourse.

Many teenage boys hear about a peculiar sexual difficulty called "penis captivus." This refers to the inability to withdraw the penis from the vagina either during or just after intercourse. An article by Egerton Y. Davis, which appeared in the *Philadelphia Medical News* of December 4, 1884, describes the condition:

When in practice at Pentonville, England, I was sent for about 11:00 p.m. by a gentleman whom, on my arriving at his house, I found in a state of great perturbation, and the story he told me was briefly as follows:

At bedtime, when going to the back kitchen to see if the house was shut up, a noise in the coachman's room attracted his attention and, going in, he discovered to his horror that the man was in bed with one of the maids. She screamed, he struggled, and they rolled out of bed together, and made frantic efforts to get apart, but without success. He was a big burly man over six feet, and she was a small woman, weighing not more than ninety pounds. She was moaning and screaming, and seemed in great agony, so that after several fruitless attempts to get them apart, he sent for me.

When I arrived, I found the man standing up and supporting the woman in his arms, and it was quite evident that his penis was tightly locked in her vagina, and any attempt to dislodge it was accompanied by much pain on the part of both. It was, indeed, a case "De cohesione in coitu." I applied water, and then ice, but ineffectively, and at last sent for chloroform, a few whiffs of which sent the woman to sleep, relaxed the spasm, and relieved the captive penis, which was swollen, livid, and in a state of semierection which did not go down for several hours, and for days the organ was extremely sore. The woman recovered rapidly, and seemed none the worse.

A frightening story—but it's a hoax, perpetuated by one of the greatest physicians of all times, Sir William Osler, using the pen name Egerton Y. Davis. Apparently, Osler wrote this case as part of a plan to embarrass another physician with whom he did not get along.

Many physicians have taken the case to be real and have perpetuated the myth within the medical profession. The lay public, having heard of this condition, have also kept the idea alive.

Helping the myth survive is the knowledge of the copulatory behavior in certain animals. The penis of canines (dogs, wolves, coyotes, etc.) has a structure called a bulbous penis. This structure, which swells when the penis is erect, contributes to the copulatory tie—the animals are literally locked together for a brief time.

Myth: Vasectomies cause impotence.

Vasectomy is currently one of the most popular forms of birth control. Approximately 500,000 vasectomies are performed annually in the United States. Many men fear that this procedure will cause impotence, and they avoid having a vasectomy even if their wives have been counseled to discontinue the use of birth control pills.

A vasectomy involves removing a portion of the tube that carries sperm away from the testicles. No part of the body involved in erections is affected. But some men have expressed concern that since the sperm produced will have nowhere to go, their bodies will become flooded with sperm. One man described himself as a potential walking sperm bank. In fact, this does not occur. New sperm are produced, but old ones die and are removed by cells that are a part of the cleansing system of the body.

Vasectomy has no negative effects on sexual performance. Following a vasectomy, there are no changes in the ease and firmness of erections, the time from vaginal penetration to ejaculation, or the force of ejaculation.

The frequency of intercourse either remains unchanged or increases. Most men and women find intercourse more pleasurable because their concern over a possible pregnancy is now eliminated. Both partners feel they have greater freedom, and many women report an increased ease in achieving orgasm.

A similar myth is that, following vasectomy, ejaculation will not occur. In fact, semen is still emitted. It is free of sperm, but there is not a significant change in the volume, color, or odor of the ejaculate.

Many surveys have been conducted among men who have had a vasectomy to determine if they are pleased with their decision. Almost all of these studies show that nearly 100 percent are well satisfied. Many men describe themselves as "sexier" following this procedure.

What to Do About Demythologizing Myths

All of the above myths may produce sufficient anxiety and impotence in the ill-informed male. While many people will find them preposterous and wonder how any educated male would subscribe to them, the fact is there are many sexually uneducated males (and females) in this country who believe in them and suffer anxiety because of them.

From what we have discussed about myths, we can see that they are based on sexual misinformation. Education in sexuality is a primary approach to overcoming myths. Readers of this book are in the process of doing just that. Becoming aware of your own acceptance of sexual myths is only a start. You must examine them and learn to dispute them. Myths are sneaky. They invade our sexual confidence when we least expect them. Learn to rewrite your myths into truthful statements. Examine your sexual scripts to see where you were involved in such faulty thinking and analyze its effect on your sexual attitudes and behaviors. Remember, just because you think you "have it" intellectually does not mean that you have begun to feel it "in your gut." Time and practice will tell. The list of myths we provided in this chapter are just a few. Look for others. They are there. Then demythologize. Then enjoy yourself!

8

SEXUAL PROBLEMS ASSOCIATED WITH IMPOTENCE

A man of sense may be in haste,
but can never be in a hurry.

—*Lord Chesterfield*

Key Points:

- Premature ejaculation and declining orgasmic intensity may be associated with impotence.
- The average time to ejaculation is simply not known.
- Trying to establish an "average time to ejaculation" may be a disservice.
- The cause of premature ejaculation is unknown.
- There are at least three treatment methods available to treat premature ejaculation.
- Decreased orgasmic intensity is commonly associated with impotence.
- Decreased orgasmic intensity is a normal part of the aging process.

Two sexual problems—premature ejaculation and declining orgasmic intensity—may be associated with or precede the onset of impotence.

Uncontrollable or premature ejaculation is a very common problem. Some believe it actually occurs more frequently than impotence.

In fact, approximately a third of all cases of impotence may be preceded by this condition, and thus it may be the most common factor associated with impotence.

Premature ejaculation, like impotence, is not a new problem. Perhaps the earliest recorded case of premature ejaculation is found in Greek mythology. Erichthonius, a mythical king of Athens, was conceived when Hephaestus, the Greek god of fire, ejaculated upon Gaea, goddess of the earth. This story was mentioned by Euripides and was recorded elsewhere in the following passage:

> Athena came to Hephaestus desirous to get arms. He, being forsaken by Aphrodite, fell in love with Athena and began to pursue her; but she fled. When he got near her with much ado (for he was lame), he attempted to embrace her: but she being a chaste virgin would not submit to him and he dropped his seed on the leg of the goddess. In disgust she wiped off the seed with wool and then threw it on the ground and Erichthonius was produced.

One consequence of premature ejaculation is that a male may feel he is not meeting his sexual responsibility, since he cannot sustain an erection long enough for his female partner to achieve an orgasm. Embarrassed, he becomes preoccupied with trying to prolong his erection prior to ejaculation. He may actually count silently or otherwise try to distract himself mentally. Or he may reduce his thrusting activity. Some men will concentrate so heavily on not ejaculating too quickly that sexual intercourse no longer is pleasurable.

To define premature ejaculation is not easy. Kinsey noted that 75 percent of males ejaculate within two minutes of penetration. Ejaculation in less than this time could be considered premature. Others have suggested that ejaculation prior to ten active thrusts constitutes this condition. Other experts in the field have defined premature ejaculation as occurring when a man cannot sustain his erection long enough for his partner to have an orgasm prior to his ejaculation at least 50 percent of the time. However, this definition is not practical, since many women are unable to achieve orgasm for reasons other than the man's rapid ejaculation.

None of the above definitions seems applicable in today's society. No one is really certain how long the sex act should last. Some feel that they are very accomplished lovers if they can pull off a "quickie"; others feel they demonstrate their masculinity by prolonging intercourse.

It is interesting that wide variations exist not only among humans but also in the animal kingdom. On the one hand, chimpanzees may complete the sexual act in sixteen seconds, while the mink may remain in the coital position for as long as eight hours. The following table demonstrates copulation time for different animals.

Duration of Copulation

Worm	4 hours
Camel	5.5 minutes
Brown bear	1–3 minutes
Mosquito	4–40 seconds
Dragonfly	23 seconds
Cat	8 seconds
Bee	2 seconds
Man	?

Different cultures also display this kind of variability. Men among the Ifugao tribe of the Philippines ejaculate almost immediately upon insertion of the penis into the vagina, while the Hopi Indians attempt to delay ejaculation for as long as possible.

Premature ejaculation varies in degree. It may be more severe for certain men than for others. In extreme cases, a male may ejaculate simply at the sight of a female's nude body or as soon as he touches his female partner. In most men, ejaculatory control increases with experience. Many teenagers, particularly in their early sexual encounters, may have little control and may even ejaculate before they can get their zipper down.

It simply isn't known how long the average male takes to ejaculate. In reality, very little is achieved by trying to arrive at an average. It will only make some men, who are actually well adjusted, seem inadequate if they find that they fall below the average, and many of these men's partners may currently be thoroughly satisfied sexually.

What causes premature ejaculation? Traditional teaching is that psychological issues are at the root of the problem. Another school of thought is that it is just another of many physical differences between people. The exact cause is not known.

There are at least three different approaches to the treatment of premature ejaculation. Reflecting the belief that the problem of premature ejaculation may be psychological in origin (and this is debatable), counseling may be recommended, either by a psychiatrist, a psychologist, or a sex therapist. It is impossible to get an accurate handle on the success rate, as various individuals claim different results.

A second approach to treatment is behavior modification. A popular example is the "stop-start" technique. The male works closely with his partner or by himself and sexual stimulation stops just before he reaches the point of ejaculation. The erection is allowed to fade and then the procedure is repeated. It is hoped that with practice ejaculatory control is improved.

The third, and most recently introduced, method is pharmacological. Several drugs designed to treat other conditions have a side effect of increasing the amount of time before ejaculation occurs. Examples are Prozac, usually used for depression, and Anafranil, normally used for obsessive-compulsive behavior. These medications are highly effective and produce the quickest results. However, there are many critics of drug therapy for premature ejaculation who believe that the cause of the problem, which they maintain to be psychological, is not being addressed.

Before embarking on any form of therapy, a man who is concerned about premature ejaculation should discuss it with his partner to see if she is sexually dissatisfied or satisfied. Some men who feel they need to do something because of what they perceive to be premature ejaculation find that no such problem exists in the partner's mind.

Is early ejaculation really abnormal? One may postulate that in the animal kingdom rapid ejaculation is really an evolutionary adaptation to ensure procreation of the various species.

DECREASED ORGASMIC INTENSITY

Many men who complain of impotence will also complain that the quality of their orgasm has decreased. This may have started before or after the onset of the problems with erection. These individuals note that the pleasurable sensation associated with ejaculation is not as great as it once was. Some lose interest in sex. Others become anxious, which may impair erectile ability.

The intensity of orgasm is dependent upon many factors. These include such variables as the setting in which sexual activity is occurring, the feeling toward the female partner, the amount of foreplay, the female's physical response to stimulation, and the amount of time that has elapsed since the previous orgasm. Some men with diabetes and others with neurological conditions such as multiple sclerosis may complain of decreased orgasmic intensity. However, it is important to appreciate, as discussed in Chapter 17, which deals with changes in sexual performance that occur with aging, that some decrease in orgasmic intensity is a normal phenomenon.

ASSESSING YOUR PROBLEM

9

THE EFFECTS OF IMPOTENCE ON THE MALE

No civilized man is completely potent.
—*Sigmund Freud*

Key Points:

- Erectile problems affect men not only in the bedroom but in many facets of their lives, including their level of self-esteem and their overall relationship with their sexual partner.
- Erectile problems can lead to self-defeating behaviors in some men, which only serve to complicate their lives.
- Erectile problems can be made worse by the intrusion of anticipatory anxiety and critical self-evaluation when men approach a potentially sexual situation.
- Erectile problems can have a ripple effect across the sexual response cycle, causing difficulties with sexual desire, arousal, orgasm, and satisfaction.

What happens when a man experiences erectile difficulties? He faces a common problem, but he does so with his own unique personality and set of circumstances. As a way of exploring the complexities of a man's sexual life, let us talk about a typical man and his experiences with this very common sexual problem. We will call him Alex. He could stand for any man reading this chapter, and parts of his experience may sound familiar to many men.

Alex is an easygoing man in his late forties. He and Sally have been married for twenty years and have three children, all doing fairly well, except for experiencing the usual trials of teenagers. Alex and Sally both have careers, and the demands on their time and energy can be taxing. Alex worries about his business, which, although successful, requires a lot of attention to stay that way. The couple get along well, except for some disagreement about the school performance of their eldest daughter, who seems to be more interested in boys and her friends than in getting serious about her future plans. The family finances are stable and the in-laws maintain a respectful distance from Alex and Sally's marital life. Alex's health is "okay" but his doctor has told him to watch his weight and blood pressure and exercise regularly. Alex would be a good neighbor to any of us. But what is going on in his sexual relationship with Sally?

Alex has always taken his sexual relationship with Sally for granted. He still loves her, and after twenty years of marriage, he is pleased that, unlike some of his friends who complain about their partners, he still finds Sally sexually attractive. Sally takes care of herself and takes pride in how she looks. While they have not experimented a lot sexually, they have their usual "sexual routine," and there are no major differences about what goes on between them in bed.

Alex has trouble pinpointing exactly when or why it started, but for the past year or so, he has noticed that his erections during intercourse with Sally are not as firm as they used to be. At times when he gets an erection it is more "bendable," and while that doesn't always interfere with entering her, "the feeling isn't like it used to be." Not that he can't get a "good" erection at other times, for example with oral sex, or with occasional masturbation, but even the desire to "get off" once in a while has diminished for him. He has begun wondering if he is slowly losing his desire for sex. The usual pattern of occasionally waking up at night or in the morning with an erection has changed too. Not that Alex worries about it, for he is far too busy with concerns about getting through the work week to pay much attention. With a busy day ahead, Alex does not have time to worry about what to do if he "wakes up with a hard-on." Sally would already be up and getting the kids ready anyway!

There are other changes too. Alex likes to please Sally and has always believed that "giving her an orgasm" is part of his sexual responsibility toward her. She can come in other ways, through oral sex or masturbation, and more recently with a vibrator. He has felt a little bit in competition with the vibrator, but many of her friends now have them, and the women are not ashamed to tell one another about their experiences. So Alex has reluctantly gone along with the "new openness" to women's sexuality. (He even has begun to feel that women are sexually superior, given all the talk about women's capability of being multiply orgasmic. Many men are busily trying to avoid being premature ejaculators.) Sally also shares Alex's notion that he is responsible for having her reach orgasm. Never mind that sometimes it takes a while for her to come.

Over the years, Alex has learned to postpone ejaculation fairly well in order to accommodate Sally. But recently he has noticed that he begins to lose some of his erection when he holds back from coming. He has had to work harder to pay attention to what he was doing—making love to his wife! Alex has also noticed at times that when his erections and arousal level diminish, he also begins to lose some of his desire for both sex and Sally. In fact, when this has happened, he has had to admit to himself that he has become bored and isn't paying attention to Sally. He is losing his energy for and interest in sex—sometimes while sex is happening! In fact, there are times when he wishes he weren't there in bed with her at all! He feels ashamed of those feelings and has begun to worry more about his erections and his sex drive. They rarely talk about their sex lives, and Alex hopes that Sally hasn't noticed the changes in his sexual performance.

Alex has begun to notice other changes too. Before these erectile difficulties, sex and "performance" were taken for granted. Now he finds himself thinking—and worrying—about them. Thoughts like "What happens if it happens again?" have begun to filter into his consciousness. Part of him knows it is silly to think this way, but Alex feels "less of a man." The word "impotence" repels him. He has told himself that some "erectile difficulties" are part of every man's life and he is not really becoming "impotent." Nevertheless, anxiety about future performance nags at him and he has begun to avoid situations with Sally that could lead to sex. He knows that sexual avoidance only buys him time, but the anxiety of "what will happen next" haunts him. He has begun to rationalize that he is getting older anyway, that his hormones are lower, that all he and Sally need is some time away from the kids. Sexual frequency has declined, and with it satisfaction with sex and with life as well. He misses his old self. Alex has begun to experience moods of sadness. Could depression be next?

Alex feels very alone in his worries. He has arrived at a place where it does not matter if the cause of the erection problems is biological, psychological, or a combination of a dozen factors. He is flooded with a sense of personal shame, failure, and guilt. He has begun to realize that he is grieving a loss. Alex shares what so many other men realize when they experience erectile difficulties and failure: loss of the ability to keep an erection is a "loss." Alex is going through a mourning process. He feels as if he has lost part of himself. Alex's experience of "loss" is an all too common emotion for many men troubled by impotence and is appreciated far too little.

WHAT IS GOING ON?

Our response to whatever happens to us in life is greatly influenced by our basic personality and total life experience. The reaction to episodes of erectile failure is no different. Even an otherwise well-adjusted man can have his confidence shaken by erectile failure. A man's response to his inability to obtain or maintain an erection can be accompanied by any number of thoughts, feelings, and behaviors that may range from mild annoyance, or even amusement, to self-doubt or despair. Blame directed at oneself or the partner is frequent, and a fragile relationship can worsen. Some men respond with self-defeating behavior such as excessive alcohol use, drug abuse, or having an affair, or even visiting prostitutes in the hope of restoring sexual functioning and confidence. Depression is common in men predisposed to mood disorders. Erectile problems cause some men to question their sexual orientation or experience shame and guilt that they have not lived up to their expected gender role. Other men begin to have mixed feelings about sexual behavior in general, feelings rooted in family, societal, or religious sex-negative messages about the body.

The nature and intensity of the man's response to erectile problems will depend on a number of factors, including the frequency and circumstances of the episodes, the status of the relationship with the sexual partner, and whether or not he has had previous bouts of impotence. Is the impotence related to a physical cause, such as a medical condition or injury? Was alcohol, medication, or drug use involved? Ignorance of sexual matters in general can be a cause. Many men are high-functioning adults in their family and professional lives but are attempting to live their sexual lives armed with an inadequate education about sexuality. Age is also a factor. The younger man may be overwhelmed with worry about performance; an older man may be panicked when the automatic erections of his youth fail to materialize. On occasion, any male can have erectile difficulties. His reaction can turn an occasional occurrence into a periodic problem. A "periodic problem" can become a chronic sexual dysfunction that in turn influences the man's life far beyond the bedroom.

We started by saying that our responses to what life deals us are in part influenced by basic personality factors. When it comes to the area of our sexual functioning, we are speaking of our sexual sense of self—our sexual self-image. Our sexual self-image is influenced by many factors, including our personal learning history, our attitudes about things sexual, and our previous sexual behaviors. It includes sexual thoughts, feelings (and feelings about those feelings), fantasies, and actions. A man's personal sex history—every man has one—will have a part to play in his response to impotence. We have discussed these notions in detail in Chapter 5, on the psychological causes of impotence, but it is important to reemphasize that when a man experiences impotence, it is his sexual self-image as well as his general self-esteem that is involved or in some way threatened. This is what is meant when people speak of the male ego being on the line. Yes, it hurts! But what a man tells himself about the problem will have a great effect on his overall and eventual response. We began this chapter with the story of Alex. If the reader puts himself into Alex's story, what would he be feeling and thinking?

PERFORMANCE ANXIETY AND SPECTATORING

The self-doubt and shame that a man can experience because of impotence (here we will use the term to refer both to occasional episodes and to chronic erectile failures) can result in significant negative and "automatic" thinking that leads to what sex therapists refer to as "performance anxiety and spectatoring." As a consequence of an instance of erectile failure, a man will often become anxious when approaching his next sexual situation. While a certain amount of anxiety is understandable, the level of anticipatory anxiety is increased if another failure is experienced. Anxiety easily intensifies and becomes panic. (There is an old saying that "anxiety" is the first time a man cannot get it up twice, and "panic" is the second time a man cannot get it up once.) This pattern tends to be repeated with each sexual opportunity. Men can worry so much in advance about failure that they are out of the game before they even get to bat. To further the analogy, even if they get up to bat they often strike out. Seeing oneself as a sexual failure increases the chances of having difficulty.

It is also important to note that too many men have exaggerated notions about what a successful or satisfying sexual experience might be, and they are most likely to increase their concern if they have an experience (notice we did not use the word "performance") that does not live up to their standards. Thus, as we stated, many men will do so much worrying ahead of time about erectile failure that their worry becomes a self-fulfilling prophecy. Remember, the penis is very sensitive to anxiety. (We are again reminded of Alex's story.)

Performance anxiety is a nuisance that can surprise both men and women when they least expect it. When the anxiety about sexual functioning becomes great enough, some men will withdraw from sexual activity as a way of avoiding failure. Unfortunately, this can result in sexless relationships if the couple's reaction to difficulties is not to engage in sexual activity at all. Sadly, many couples do not seek assistance when help may be readily available.

Spectatoring is the twin of performance anxiety. While sex is a "participant sport" for most people, for some men sexual activity becomes a closely watched, critically observed event. Spectatoring means watching oneself do it! It leads to observing and interrupting the flow of sexual activity by, for example, wondering "How am I doing? . . . Is it hard enough? . . . What is my partner thinking? . . . It's okay now, but maybe I should hurry before I lose it again. . . . What will my partner think if I get soft before she even comes? What if I come too soon?" Both performance anxiety and spectatoring usually occur as a result of erectile failure, and both need therapeutic intervention.

THE SEXUAL RESPONSE CYCLE

A helpful way to understand how men respond to erectile difficulties is to place the problem within the overall sexual response cycle. Traditionally, approaches to understanding human sexual response focused on how arousal eventually led to orgasm. While understanding this mechanism helps to clarify what happens to the body during sexual activity, it does not clarify what is going on in the person as a sexual being. A new term, DAVOS, was introduced by Dr. Harold Lief, a pioneering sex therapist, and it will serve as a guide throughout this book to put sexual functioning into an integrated perspective. DAVOS will also help to place into perspective some of the possible effects of impotence in the overall sexual functioning in men, as well as the interplay of the elements of sexual response in both men and women.

DESIRE
AROUSAL
VASOCONGESTION
ORGASM
SATISFACTION

Desire is where sexual interest and response begin. Dr. Harold Lief and Dr. Helen Kaplan, also a prominent sex therapist, made a considerable contribution to the study of human sexuality when they introduced desire as a major component of sexual response. We know it when it is present as well as when it is absent. It cannot be faked, but it can be kindled. Problems of sexual desire are a common complaint of many men and women in today's busy world.

Arousal is the psychological and physiological perception that a person is getting turned on sexually. Arousal has certain physical signs that make us aware of our sexual feeling. It is necessary to maintain the rest of the sexual response cycle. Both desire and arousal can be inhibited by anxiety, and problems in these areas can be major components in the cause and treatment of sexual dysfunctions.

Vasocongestion is the erection response in men and the parallel response in women of vaginal lubrication and genital swelling.

Orgasm is experienced as a total body response in both sexes and is usually associated with, but is still separate from, ejaculation in men. Orgasm and ejaculation are so closely related that men tend to use the term "orgasm" to describe the overall experience and sensation, although the two can be desynchronized (i.e., there can be ejaculation without orgasm and orgasm without ejaculation).

Satisfaction is a subjective state that describes the person's evaluation of sexual activity as being good or worthwhile. Since it is a subjective state, the level of satisfaction that is experienced is sensitive to many variables that are related to intimacy, sexual sharing, pleasure, and a host of values that are used to judge the quality of an experience. The level of satisfaction need not be directly related to the actual physical enjoyment of the sexual activity, and it may involve gender differences. For example, men tend to equate "good sex" with erections and orgasms, while many women claim to be satisfied even though they did not have an orgasm. Conversely, some orgasmic women may not be satisfied with sex because of trouble in the relationship. In the final analysis, sex therapists recognize the subjective nature of sexual satisfaction and consider good sex to be what you and your partner feel good about afterwards.

We can examine the DAVOS model to explore some of the influences that impotence could have elsewhere in the sexual response cycle. A man who is experiencing erection problems would be experiencing dysfunction in the categories of arousal and vasocongestion, whether the cause was physical or psychological. Something is inhibiting his ability to gain or maintain an erection. What effect could the impotence have on the rest of the cycle? We pointed out earlier that anticipatory anxiety causes concern about future sexual functioning. ("Will I be able to do it this time?") Problems in one area of sex can lead to difficulties in another. It is a small shift for a man to move from worrying about getting an erection to losing desire for sex altogether. For a single male, without a regular sex partner, it often is the case that sexual abstinence is the route taken to avoid further embarrassment and frustration.

For those men who don't try to protect their self-esteem by choosing abstinence, it is a daunting task to continue attempting intercourse.

Whether he has a regular partner or not, a man troubled by impotence worries about his level of arousal. The arousal level, vitally important in achieving and maintaining an erection, can easily be inhibited by anxiety. The result can be a loss of whatever erection has occurred. Orgasm can be affected by the same mechanisms. A man may ejaculate very quickly or have difficulty ejaculating at all. For him, satisfaction may become a thing of the past, regardless of the reassurance of a sympathetic partner. We are reminded that responses throughout the DAVOS cycle can represent a cascading effect in which the original problem of impotence overflows into the other areas of the sexual cycle.

We have mentioned that what often happens in cases of impotence is that the man and his partner abstain from sexual activity altogether, and this can lead to overall relationship difficulties. For one thing, the partners are deprived of the closeness and intimacy that sexual contact brings. This is especially true if the couple's pattern of sexual behavior is limited mainly to intercourse. If they believe that sex means "intercourse or nothing," the options for ongoing closeness are limited. The resulting stress on the relationship can stir up other unresolved problems, bringing to the fore long-smoldering issues that complicate matters even more. The struggle for adjustment may be waged with dysfunctional and inadequate ways of communicating and relating. Such maladaptive coping mechanisms did not work before and will not work under these circumstances. Past traumas in the relationship or from the history of either partner may surface as a result of the stress. Some couples fight back by trying harder to make sex work, but anxiety and repeated failure discourage them. This scenario sounds bleak, and for many men with erection problems it can be. The work required to return to sexual health is well worth the effort.

WHERE DO YOU STAND? A QUICK EVALUATION

Just as we saw that the DAVOS model can help us better understand the pattern of sexual response, another model can help in evaluating how other areas of psychological and social functioning are affected by impotence.

Psychologist Arnold A. Lazarus, the developer of "multimodal therapy," explains that a person can be described by a number of categories or "modalities" that collectively are described by the acronym BASIC ID. A person's functioning can be outlined as follows:

*B*EHAVIOR (positive or negative)
*A*FFECT (feelings, e.g., anxiety or depression)
*S*ENSATIONS (bodily, including sexual)
*I*MAGERY (mental pictures or representations)
*C*OGNITIONS (thoughts, positive or negative)

*I*NTERPERSONAL RELATIONS (relating to others)
*D*RUGS (medications or physical conditions)

Using the BASIC ID to run a self-profile is rather easy. As an example, in each category or modality, a man can ask himself what specific *behaviors* he would like to increase or decrease (e.g., be more sexually assertive, be less avoidant); what *feelings* trouble him the most (e.g., anger, sadness); what *sensations* he would like to increase or decrease (e.g., be more tuned in to sexual sensations); what *thoughts* he would like to decrease or increase (e.g., thinking of self as sexual failure, having more sexual confidence); what *mental pictures or images* trouble him or he would like to have or change (e.g., from dysfunctional sex to healthy sexual functioning); how his *interpersonal relationships* are going (e.g., what effect impotence has on relating to the sexual partner); and what his general health status is (does it contribute to and/or is it a consequence of the sexual problem?).

A man with erectile difficulties can take his response to impotence and run it through the modalities of the BASIC ID. What he will find is just how much his erectile problems are influencing other aspects of his psychic and personal life. For instance, let's say that John Doe, who has been having recurrent erectile failure, is avoiding sexual situations (*behavior*), is feeling depressed and angry (*affect*); has developed headaches and a nervous stomach (*sensations*); has images of failed attempts at sex, with little vision for future improvement (*imagery*); experiences constant thoughts of low self-esteem and failure (*cognitions*); is short-tempered at work and at home (*interpersonal relationships*); and is drinking too much and has neglected his usual exercise routine (*drugs*).

There are many John Does out there with a similar BASIC ID profile. We saw some similarities when we discussed Alex's problems with his sexuality. But the difficulties can be turned around. The boundaries between the different BASIC ID modalities are permeable, so that a change in one area can positively influence the others. For example, a sexual success (we will also always take luck when it presents itself) can have positive ripple effects across the BASIC ID so that changes in behavior, mood, self-image, positive self-thoughts, etc., can all take place. There is always hope. Change and improvement can take place. Sexual health is just around the corner.

10

WHEN YOU SEEK HELP, WHAT KIND OF EVALUATION SHOULD YOU HAVE?

That man to me seems to possess but one idea,
and that is a wrong one.

—*Samuel Johnson*

Key Points:

- Some disagreement exists within the medical profession as to what constitutes an appropriate evaluation for impotence.
- At minimum, a complete medical and *sexual* history, a physical examination, and basic blood tests should be carried out. The extent of further testing will depend upon the results.
- The patient's goals should be considered before pursuing further studies.
- Every impotent male does not require every test available!

What constitutes a proper evaluation for a male with impotence? It is the subject of much debate among doctors. Some of the differences of opinion and the confusions that exist, even among experts, are due to a revision of our understanding of the causes of erectile insufficiency, as well as new treatment options. Until recently, it was believed that the cause of erectile insufficiency in 90 percent of the cases was psychological as opposed to physical. As more knowledge and a better understanding of the mechanism of erection evolved, the pendulum began to swing, so that by the 1980s, many experts felt that at least half the cases of impotence were due to physical causes. In this decade, the pendulum continues to swing to the extent that many doctors, particularly urologists, believe that approximately 90 percent of the cases have physical causes. The fact is that no one knows for sure what percentage of impotence is psychological in origin and what percentage is due to physical causes. In truth, in many, if not most, cases, there are both physical and psychological factors contributing to the problem. The difficulty of separating psychological and physical factors in any illness was appreciated years ago by Samuel Butler:

> *BODY and MIND. We shall never get straight till we leave off trying to separate these two things. Mind is not a thing at all or, if it is, we know nothing about it. It is a function of the body. The body is not a thing at all or, if it is, we know nothing about it. It is a function of the mind.*

A consensus panel from the National Institutes of Health states that:

> *Psychosocial factors are important in all forms of erectile dysfunction. Careful attention to these issues and attempts to relieve sexual anxieties should be a part of all the therapeutic intervention for all patients.*

In recent years, two factors have emerged that augment the debate over what constitutes a proper evaluation. The first is the introduction of less invasive forms of treatment for impotence, and the second is the change from traditional health insurance to managed care plans.

Use of vacuum constriction devices, self-injections, small pellets that can be inserted in the tip of the penis, and oral medication have raised the question of whether or not it is really important to know the cause of the erectile insufficiency. Some health care providers take the position that before any form of treatment is offered one should know what is causing the impotence. Others, including those whose responsibility it is to hold down the cost of health care, argue that since the patient is only complaining of not being able to get an erection, you have treated him adequately when you give him something to produce an erection, even without knowing the cause of his problem.

In the past, evaluation consisted of a complete medical and sexual history, a physical examination, and appropriate blood tests such as blood count, cholesterol level, and serum testosterone. Patients also had a psychological evaluation, meeting with a psychologist, psychiatrist, or sex therapist and/or completing certain written psychological tests. Then, as a more thorough understanding of the erection process developed and modern medical technology progressed, an assessment of the blood flow to the penis was added to the list of diagnostic tests.

Evaluations still vary. Some doctors insist upon a comprehensive evaluation. Others do not. Now that less invasive treatments have become available, many patients will receive treatment without any significant evaluation. Whether this constitutes good medical care can be debated. Usually it is prudent to know the cause of a medical problem before treating it.

Most health care professionals agree that obtaining a medical and sexual history and performing a relevant physical examination are almost always appropriate. A debate centers around whether blood tests are needed, and if so, which ones. Disagreement intensifies if invasive tests are suggested.

WHICH TESTS MAY BE RECOMMENDED?

In addition to taking a patient's medical and sexual history, performing a physical examination, and obtaining blood tests, other tests may be advised, some of which are listed below.

Erotic video testing

This test is just what the title implies. A patient watches an erotic video while measurements are made of changes in the expansion of the penis and the degree of rigidity.

After small delicate bands are placed around the base and tip of the penis, the patient is left in privacy while a machine records changes in measurement. If a solid erection develops during erotic video testing, it is clear that the cause of erectile insufficiency is psychological rather than physical.

Tests to assess blood flow

Duplex ultrasonography. Since blood flow into the penis is essential for achieving a solid erection, it is important to measure the flow of blood into the penis and to see whether it is stored appropriately to allow expansion and rigidity. One of the most accurate of these tests is duplex sonography. A drug that induces blood flow is injected into the erectile tissue of the penis through a fine needle. This stimulates an erection. Ultrasound is then used to measure the diameter of the arteries and the velocity of blood flow inside the erectile compartments.

Penile arteriography. In this test, dye is injected in order to visualize the arteries that carry blood to the penis. Any point of blockage may be identified. In addition, if the blood drains too rapidly from the penis, this may be noted as well. This condition is called "venous leak." Penile arteriography provides a "picture" of the blood vessels in the penis.

Dynamic infusion corpora cavernosometry (DICC). In simple terms, an erection may be thought of as a hydraulic system in which fluid (blood) must flow rapidly into the erection chambers of the penis and not leak out prematurely (venous leakage). DICC measures the rise in pressure in the penis and helps determine if it is sufficient to create rigidity. If blood leaks out of the erection chambers prematurely, this will be detected. While penile arteriography provides a picture of the blood vessels in the penis, DICC reveals pressure changes.

Both penile arteriography and DICC testing are invasive procedures. They are generally not recommended unless a patient and his urologist are prepared to proceed with surgical correction of either reduced inflow into the penis or too rapid drainage from the penis. Before consenting to these tests, the patient should have a frank discussion with his physician about what treatment recommendation will follow. This is particularly important since the results of surgery to improve the blood flow are generally not good unless the problem is due to a localized or segmental blockage. Similarly, the long-term results for correction of venous leakage have been disappointing.

NPT testing

In some cases, nocturnal penis tumescence (NPT) testing will be recommended. This is usually when it is not clear whether the impotence is due to physical or psychological factors. Sleep research reveals that there are regularly recurring periods of sleep associated with a characteristic brain wave pattern and with rapid eye movement (REM). REM sleep is also associated with dreaming. It is at these times that erections take place. REM sleep normally occurs approximately four to five times a night and is associated with a strong erection which lasts approximately 15 to 25 minutes each time.

Erections during REM sleep occur from birth to old age. During adolescence, 90 percent of REM sleep is associated with strong erections, whereas between the ages of forty and fifty, only 66 percent of REM sleep is accompanied by erections. In addition, the length of time that erections last declines as age increases.

NPT testing may be conducted in a sleep laboratory, or the patient may be sent home with a portable monitor. Two small bands, one placed around the base of the penis and the other around the tip, are linked to a recording device that monitors expansion and rigidity for an eight-hour period. Usually two or three nights of testing are required. The test is painless.

The theory behind NPT testing is that if a male demonstrates sufficient expansion and rigidity while asleep, the blood flow and nerves supplying the penis are normal and the patient's problem is psychological. However, not all experts agree on the utility of NPT testing. If the patient is tested on a home monitor and no erections develop, a valid question arises as to whether the patient ever slept deeply enough to enter REM sleep. (In a sleep laboratory, brain waves are monitored and it is possible to tell whether the patient ever reached the appropriate depth of sleep.) A second criticism is that the NPT monitor only records expansion and makes an indirect computation for rigidity. Some experts feel that this measure of rigidity (radial) does not really reflect the true pressure that it would take to make the penis bend (axial rigidity). In addition, some experts believe that erections that occur while asleep are not the same as sexual erections. This is based upon the evaluation of patients who appear to have no physical or psychological problems causing their impotence. These patients may achieve excellent erections when tested at night but cannot achieve an erection during a sexual encounter.

Other factors can confuse the issue. Emotional states have been demonstrated to adversely affect nighttime erectile activity. Such states include anxiety, depression, and severe loss of libido. Various medicines may also inhibit nighttime erections. Finally, the quality of nighttime erections changes with aging. Older men may experience a decline in the number of erections as well as in rigidity of the penis.

Home monitor results should not be used as the only criterion to determine whether the erectile problem is "psychological" or "physical." Rather, they should be regarded as one piece of data that must be correlated with the complete medical and sexual history, physical examination, and blood test results.

OUR RECOMMENDATION

Every male who complains of impotence does *not* require every diagnostic test currently available. Each case must be considered individually.

The decision as to which tests to order depends on several major factors. The first is the findings from the medical and sexual history, physical examination, and usually blood tests. If the treating physician, psychologist, or sex therapist is confident that he or she can establish an accurate diagnosis or that treatment is appropriate without a specific diagnosis after the history, physical examination, and laboratory results, no further tests may be required for patients who favor relatively noninvasive treatment such as a vacuum device or one of the various types of pharmacological treatment—injections, pellet, or pill. For patients whose problem is clearly psychological in origin, counseling or psychotherapy is usually appropriate.

The second factor is the patient's own goals. Is he intent on knowing the cause of his potency problem or is he really more interested in just receiving treatment so that he will be able to perform?

Without being dogmatic, it should be emphasized that prior to any form of therapy a minimal evaluation should include a thorough medical and sexual history, physical examination, and often screening blood tests. The following case study demonstrates this point.

> *H. F., a fifty-eight-year-old male, experienced difficulty in achieving erections. He told his family physician that this problem seemed to be of gradual onset over the past one or two years. The problem seemed to be persistent and progressive. The patient was an executive running a high-powered business and was under considerable stress in his job. His eating habits were poor and he continued to smoke one pack of cigarettes per day. He described himself as a poor sleeper. Another source of stress was a child who had recently dropped out of college and seemed to have no direction in life.*

From this history one might conclude that the patient's failure to achieve erections was due to psychological stress both in his workplace and at home. However, this patient, when evaluated, was thought to have poor blood flow to the penis. While the psychological factors are important, it is the reduced blood flow that may have been more significant. Why is this so? Because poor blood flow may be occurring in other organs, particularly the heart and brain. This particular patient is at a higher risk for a heart attack or stroke even though he has not yet shown any symptoms that might prompt him to see his family doctor or cardiologist. In short, his impotence should sound an alarm that he needs a thorough vascular evaluation.

Getting to know the patient will usually help in selecting the most appropriate form of therapy. In addition, choosing the correct dosage of certain medications used to treat impotence is in part dependent on the presence or absence of other diseases, such as diabetes or liver or kidney insufficiency.

If a careful *sexual* history is not taken, the patient may be given treatment for a condition he does not have. For example, some men confuse impotence with premature ejaculation, a low level of sexual desire, decreased orgasmic intensity, or a prolonged period of time after ejaculation during which it is impossible to ejaculate again. Thus, an incorrect diagnosis may lead to the wrong treatment.

11

SELF-EVALUATION FOR THE MALE:
YOU BE THE DOCTOR

"Know thyself" is indeed a weighty admonition. But
in this, as in science, the difficulties are discovered
only by those who set their hands to it. We must push
against a door to find out whether it is bolted or not.
— *Montaigne*

Key Points:

The most important step in determining the underlying cause of
impotence is obtaining an accurate medical and sexual history.
  Relevant questions fall into four areas:
- Sexual function
- Relationship issues
- Past medical history
- Personal history
  If you are having a problem, answering the questions will be
very helpful.

Any male who is impotent will profit from an honest analysis of his
personal situation, and a female will gain insight into her partner's difficulty through this analysis. The following questions, if they are carefully
considered, will allow a male or female to put the problem in perspective. The information that is collected will be very valuable to any physi-

cian, psychologist, or counselor who seeks to aid the male having sexual difficulties. It is much easier to answer these questions in an honest and realistic fashion if one does so in the quiet, unpressured setting of the home rather than in the doctor's office, where one may feel rushed.

An interpretation of each question appears below it.

FUNCTION QUESTIONS

Question 1: What bothers you about your sexual functioning? That is, what is your problem?

1. Low sexual desire in general
2. Low sexual desire for my partner
3. Not feeling aroused (turned on)
4. Not getting an erection sufficient for intercourse
5. Not keeping an erection
6. Not having an orgasm (climax), even though I feel aroused
7. Ejaculating too quickly (coming too fast)
8. Having an orgasm that lacks intensity
9. Having an orgasm but not being able to ejaculate
10. Pain during sex

Interpretation of Question 1

Answering the question should get to the heart of your problem. Some men are able to have an erection but cannot ejaculate or have orgasm. Some men can erect and ejaculate but experience a decline in the intensity of the orgasm. Others are able to ejaculate and have orgasm with a soft penis. Some men can attain an erection but not sustain it in order to penetrate and complete the sex act. Others can erect and penetrate but ejaculate too quickly to satisfy themselves or their partner. Some men will experience pain in the genitalia with sexual activity. Having defined your problem, let's determine the cause.

Question 2: Have you ever had an erection?

Interpretation of Question 2

If you have never had an erection sufficient for sexual performance in your life, you are suffering from "primary" impotence. This suggests either a serious physical problem or a deep-seated emotional one that will require professional counseling.

The vast majority of impotent men have "secondary" impotence—that is, they have previously had satisfactory erections permitting intercourse.

Question 3: When is the last time you had what you would consider a complete, normal erection followed by ejaculation?

Interpretation of Question 3

It is important to estimate the time of onset of your difficulty. Impotence of short duration is very often psychologically related to a specific event or has a physical cause such as beginning a new medication or having gone through a surgical procedure. Impotence that is of a longer duration and has come on slowly but progressively usually has a physical cause such as poor blood flow.

Question 4: Are you able to achieve an erection with masturbation? If so, what percent of a full erection do you get?

Interpretation of Question 4

Being able to achieve a full erection with self-stimulation or that provided by your partner indicates normal blood and nerve supply to your penis. Being able to become erect with masturbation but not for intercourse usually indicates a psychological problem.

Question 5: When you awaken during the night or in the morning, what percent of a full erection have you seen in the last few months?

Interpretation of Question 5

Erections that occur during the night are indicative of normal nerve and blood flow to the penis. As previously noted, every normal male will have three to five erections at night, each lasting 20 to 25 minutes. These are not generally appreciated by the male (although they may be by his partner) because they only occur at a certain depth of sleep. The erection that is noted upon awakening, contrary to popular opinion, is not due to a full bladder. It is a reflection of one of the normal erections occurring during rapid-eye movement sleep. The presence of these erections is a very favorable sign and often points to a psychological cause.

Question 6: If you read erotic material or see an erotic movie, what percent of a full erection do you usually get?

Interpretation of Question 6

An erection brought about by an erotic thought or visual stimulus is initiated in the brain. This is a very favorable sign and again is indicative of normal function of the nerve and blood supply to the penis, suggesting a psychological cause.

Question 7: Are you able to get a good firm erection at some times and not at others?

Interpretation of Question 7

If you get a good-quality erection at any time that is sufficient to complete the act of intercourse, yet at other times you are impotent, it is quite likely that your difficulty is psychological.

Question 8: Does erectile difficulty occur only with a certain partner?

Interpretation of Question 8

If you are impotent only with a certain partner but can perform successfully with someone else, there is not likely to be any physical problem causing impotence. (This is *not* a suggestion that you try multiple partners, particularly if you are married.) It does, however, suggest that sex therapy or marriage counseling should be considered.

RELATIONSHIP QUESTIONS

Question 9: Does your partner know that you are seeking help and have come for an evaluation?

Interpretation of Question 9

If an impotent male has discussed the problem with his partner, it indicates good communication. Treatment is more likely to be successful if his partner is aware.

Question 10: Is your partner supportive of your seeking help?

Interpretation of Question 10

Men who have supportive partners are more likely to experience a quick recovery. Men whose partners are not supportive are generally angry and resentful, which does not help the healing process.

Question 11: Do you find your partner sexually attractive?

Interpretation of Question 11

Men who are no longer "turned on" by their partner are more likely to experience impotence. Males who do not accept the normal changes in a partner's body that occur with aging may have unrealistic expectations and desires.

Question 12: Has your sexual problem caused any of the following difficulties in your relationship?

1. "Chilly" atmosphere in the house
2. Less overall communication
3. Avoidance of specific topics like sex
4. More arguing
5. Withdrawal from family members or friends
6. Less trust in my partner
7. Less trust in me by my partner
8. Doing fewer activities together

Interpretation of Question 12

Like a stone cast in the water, a sexual problem may have a ripple effect upon a couple's entire relationship. Arguing, avoidance, distrust, frustration, and discouragement or depression are more likely to occur in either or both individuals.

Question 13: Do you or does your partner usually initiate sexual activity?

Interpretation of Question 13

If one partner always initiates sexual activity, it may be indicative of widely differing levels of interest in sex or reflect negative feelings about the relationship. In an ideal world, each partner may initiate sex at different times depending upon urge, interest level, and a desire to satisfy each other.

Question 14: Do you feel it is important that your female partner climax during every episode of intercourse? Do you feel that all sexual encounters must include intercourse?

Interpretation of Question 14

If you feel that you must guarantee your female partner has an orgasm during *every* sexual encounter or that you must achieve sexual penetration and vigorous thrusting, you may be placing unrealistic demands on yourself, which may lead to sexual failure.

PAST MEDICAL HISTORY QUESTIONS

Question 15: Do you have or have you had in the past any of the following?

1. High blood pressure
2. Heart disease
3. Heart attack
4. Diabetes
5. Thyroid gland disease
6. Testicular disease
7. Multiple sclerosis
8. Parkinson's disease
9. Other neurological disease
10. Stroke
11. Kidney disease
12. Cancer

Interpretation of Question 15

Any of these illnesses may indicate a general medical problem that can cause difficulties with sexual functioning. It is important that your physician, psychologist, or counselor be fully aware of such problems. All of these may indicate an underlying physical cause of impotence.

Question 16: Have you had any of the following surgical procedures?

1. Removal of the prostate
2. Removal of the bladder
3. Rectal or colon surgery
4. Cardiac bypass
5. Disk surgery
6. Vascular surgery of the legs or major blood vessels

Interpretation of Question 16

Any of these operations may indicate a physical cause for your impotence because of an impairment of blood flow or nerve function.

Question 17: What medications do you take?

Interpretation of Question 17

Commonly prescribed medicines such as antidepressants, blood pressure pills, sedatives, hormones, drugs for peptic ulcer, and over-the-counter cold medications can contribute to erectile failure. You should review your medications with your physician. However, keep in mind that most men who take these medications do not experience impotence.

Question 18: Did your sexual problem begin soon after taking a new drug?

Interpretation of Question 18

If you can document in your mind that your difficulty began soon after starting a new medication, this may be a very important point. It suggests that this drug may be causing or contributing to your problem.

Question 19: Have you ever had an erection that lasted several hours?

Interpretation of Question 19

A past history of an excessively prolonged erection (usually more than four to six hours) may prevent future erections. This is due to damage caused to the erectile tissue, which is generally not reversible.

PERSONAL HISTORY QUESTIONS

Question 20: Do you smoke, abuse alcohol, use illicit drugs, or have high cholesterol? Do you believe that you are not in good physical condition?

Interpretation of Question 20

Any of these factors, smoking, elevated cholesterol, abusing alcohol, or failing to exercise, may contribute to difficulties with sexual functioning.

Question 21: Do your legs ache when you walk more than a few blocks?

Interpretation of Question 21

Poor blood supply to the pelvis and the legs, which is usually caused by atherosclerosis, may indicate poor blood flow to the penis, which may cause impotence.

Question 22: If you have heart disease or have had a heart attack, are you fearful of dying during intercourse or is your partner fearful of having sex with you for this reason?

Interpretation of Question 22

Anxiety following a heart attack may keep you from resuming a normal sexual life. If your partner has major concerns, she may be unwilling to participate in sex for fear of precipitating a heart attack or stroke. Many men who have suffered from such an illness and whose partner refrains from sex out of concern for them often misinterpret her restraint as a lack of interest.

These questions and your answers are intended only as a framework to help you understand your problem and to aid a professional sex counselor or a physician in managing your case. Many men who answer these questions will figure out for themselves whether the cause of their impotence is likely to be psychological or physical, or both. Most are relieved once they have taken a step toward understanding their own diagnosis. Once you pinpoint your difficulty, you will have a better understanding of diagnostic tests or treatment that your physician may recommend.

TREATING YOUR PROBLEM

12

TREATING PSYCHOLOGICAL CAUSES OF IMPOTENCE

The man who removes a mountain begins by carrying away small stones.

—*Chinese proverb*

Key Points:

- Successful treatment of erectile dysfunction often requires a combination of medical and psychological intervention.
- What is "normal" sexual functioning can vary from one man to another.
- All successful treatment begins with a proper evaluation, including a sexual history, a clear understanding of the specific sexual problem, and an appropriate medical examination.
- Treatment should be specific to the problems. Not every man requires the same intervention.
- The role of foreplay is very important and is more than technique. It is a form of intimate communication between partners.
- Self-help exercises can be very helpful in overcoming erectile difficulties.

BACK TO BASICS: START AT THE BEGINNING

We have been making an assumption that sexual functioning is a natural process and enjoying sexual health means allowing the individual to experience his sexuality without interference of ignorance, coercion, guilt, shame, disease, or dysfunction. It is true, however, that individual men vary in their subjective and physiological response, and there is no *one* way for a man to respond sexually. For example, the time or stimulation required to obtain an erection may vary, as may the amount of time before ejaculation occurs. What is "normal" is really a range of behavior or responses. What one man sees as normal may be seen as a problem by another, and vice versa.

It is also true that men can interfere with their own sexual and erectile response in a number of ways. We know how negative thoughts, performance anxiety, inappropriate circumstances for sex, and partner conflicts can compromise a man's chances of obtaining and maintaining erections. We have emphasized the role of understanding the sexual response cycle with the acronym DAVOS, and how erections flow from a nurtured desire that leads to arousal and the sense of being "turned on." We noted that erections tend to "take care of themselves" if we can unlock the barriers to desire and arousal in ourselves and our partners. We have made a point of focusing on pleasure rather than on performance goals as a way of almost paradoxically achieving the desired level of arousal that leads to good erections. Sexual encounters begin and end with pleasure. Pleasure leads to satisfaction, and satisfaction provides the motivation for continuing and repeating sexual expressions with one's partner.

TREATMENT: WHO NEEDS IT?

One of the criticisms of the traditional or "Freudian" approach to psychotherapy was that, to some extent, patients received the same type of treatment approach regardless of the complaint. Our popular culture is used to seeing the image, often presented with humor, of the patient "on the couch" while the therapist patiently listens, sometimes for years! Of course, many people have been and still are very much helped with an insight-oriented approach to understanding personal problems. The field of psychotherapy has evolved over the years, as have other avenues of approach, and it is recognized by mental health practitioners that not everyone requires or benefits from long-term insight-oriented therapy. Psychotherapy today is marked by greater flexibility and eclecticism. Learning from books such as this one is an example of an educational and informational approach—bibliotherapy. Not every erectile difficulty requires the same treatment, or the same level of intensity of intervention. Some erectile problems require only brief therapeutic attention, while others may need considerable effort to treat effectively.

WHAT IS BEING TREATED?

Nick is a forty-year-old man who is quite happy in his second marriage. His wife, Claire, is a good mother to their two children and runs her own successful business. She is all he could ask for—except sexually. Claire is a bit inhibited sexually, and while Nick thinks she has an attractive figure, she is very self-conscious about her body image. Of course, Claire has gained some weight over the past few years—it runs in her family—but she is attractive and loving. Nick, too, has put on a few pounds.

Nick has recently recovered from a mild heart attack, something unusual for a man his age. He is chronic worrier and has always paid strict attention to details. He even focuses on the details in the way he approaches Claire for sex. He has noticed that his erections just are not what they used to be. Nick confided in his best friend, who reminded Nick that his doctor had told him he was fine and not to worry about having sex. Nick is beginning to think that maybe he is just getting older (at forty?). He also knows that he is a bit turned off by Claire's weight gain. But having gained weight himself, he could never mention this to her. Besides, he really loves her, and that is all that matters. What to do about the decline of his sexual performance? Should he seek help for himself, or for the two of them, and if so, with what kind of therapist?

For men like Nick there are a number of options available for the psychological treatment of erectile problems. They range from cognitive-behavioral therapy models to more formal long-term insight-oriented treatment. The treatment that is offered can very much depend on the therapeutic orientation of the therapist. Some therapists prefer to work within a traditional model, while others are more eclectic and flexible in their approach to treating sexual dysfunction. While a man seeking assistance might prefer one treatment approach to another, it is important that he feel comfortable and at ease with whatever therapist he chooses.

It is not unusual today to see treatment that includes medical or pharmaceutical intervention in combination with counseling techniques and modalities such as individual or couples therapy. Even with the advent of medical intervention for erection difficulties, men must still relate positively to their sexual partners, who will continue to remain an integral part of the sexual equation. Medical intervention alone, without paying attention to the effects that sexual dysfunction has had on the relationship, may result in limited success and treatment that is truly incomplete.

Sex is never simple. Neither is treatment. First of all, what are we treating? Let us consider our friend Nick. Are we treating an erection? An individual male? A relationship? A couple's or family's system? A psychological reaction to a medical condition? Are we correcting a pathological condition or offering growth in sexual potential? What is the goal? Is it the restoration of "normal functioning"? Does this presume there is a "normal" erectile capacity out there for every man to achieve? Does he either achieve that or fail? And once potency is restored, is everything okay? What about individual differences in sexual interest and "performance"? Is it simply a matter of improving technique? Does just decreasing anxiety and enhancing performance run the risk of sacrificing sexual intimacy for sexual technique? Is having a good erection all that matters? If something is "broken," does fixing it cure the "problem?" Does adequate functioning mean more than just having an erection? When is treatment successful?

It seems we have many questions that may require different answers for different people. We said that sex is never simple.

Although erectile failure may be the common complaint of a man seeking psychological treatment, not every man has the same set of life circumstances, needs, or goals. Therapy begins with (1) an adequate assessment of the man's complaint or problem, including the need for medical evaluation; (2) understanding the possible causes as well as the variables that serve to maintain the problem; (3) the realistic setting of treatment goals; (4) a treatment plan to achieve those goals that is specific to the problem and circumstances while also being flexible in using whatever interventions and treatment modalities might be indicated. The therapeutic journey may be short or long. There may be surprises along the way. But treatment is always an opportunity for growth and overall improvement and enhancement of both sexual functioning and the emotional quality of life. Above all, therapy is educational.

OPENING QUESTIONS

In the previous chapter we presented a series of self-evaluation questions for men about the status of their erectile functioning. The questions covered a number of areas that would commonly be explored by a urologist or primary physician. In this section, which deals with sex therapy, we will be considering many of those self-evaluation questions about erectile functioning, but from a much more integrated, detailed, focused, and psychologically minded view. A sex therapist gathers information in an attempt to understand and clarify the sexual problem. The goal is to identify the possible causes of the erection problems; the variables that might be contributing to the continuance of the problem; the possible existence of other sexual, relationship, or personality problems; the suitability of the man (and, if indicated, his partner) for treatment; the need for possible further medical or psychological testing or consultation; and the treatment plan that could assist the man in returning to healthy sexual functioning. Throughout the remainder of this section, readers will find it helpful, and thought-provoking, to ask themselves the questions that the sex therapist is pursuing. Let's go!

Just how does the man see his problem? How does he experience it? Is the erection problem life-long—that is, has he never had an erection in either a sexual or nonsexual situation? Has the onset of the erectile difficulty been a gradual process, or is it related to a specific episode that later continued into a pattern of failure? Is it situational? Or has he had erections, but never sufficient enough for penetration in sexual contact? Or has he been able to penetrate his partner in one way but not another, that is, vaginally, orally, or anally? Has he been able to get an erection after adequate stimulation and been able to penetrate, only to lose the erection after a short period of time, varying with circumstances or partner? Can he have a good erection, for example, with masturbation, but not with intercourse? Or with oral sex, but not with intercourse? With vaginal intercourse, but not with oral sex? Does he wake up at night or in the morning with an erection? Is the erectile difficulty related to another sexual problem such as rapid (premature) ejaculation? (Chronic premature ejaculation may lead to erectile difficulties as an adaptation to avoiding disappointment during intercourse.) Are there partner issues that determine the state of his erection? For example, poor erections or impotence with his regular sex partner, but no problems with a new or novel partner? Is the relationship with the current sexual partner problematic? Are there specific or unusual circumstances required for erections?

Does he need certain types of sexual stimulation, circumstances, or fantasies in order to obtain an erection? For example, is he involved in what many people would consider "kinky" or "perverted" (therapists use the term "paraphiliac") sexual activities that he needs to provide arousal and gratification? Can this same man function with a "straight partner in straight sex"? His problem with sex may be more than just one of adequate sexual functioning. Does the medical history reveal any direct or indirect indications that could contribute to erectile failure? (Certain conditions such as diabetes, or medication side effects, may interfere with erections.) Is the impotence related to drug, alcohol, or tobacco use? (Many men refuse to realize the effects of these substances on their erectile capacity, especially as they get older.)

If the man is in a committed relationship, what is the relationship history? How healthy is the relationship? How long have sexual problems existed? What stresses are on the relationship? Are there any areas of unresolved anger or hostility? Are there "secrets" present in the relationship that need to be addressed before sex therapy can begin? If these "secrets" are ignored, are they likely to undermine treatment? (Perhaps individual consultations with the therapist would be necessary before initiating couples therapy.) Is the man (and is his partner) motivated for treatment? If the man is without a partner, he will have to examine the circumstances under which he attempts to meet partners, the strength of his interpersonal skills, and how these factors may influence his erectile failure. Performance anxiety abounds in singles bars! The single male, whether he be bachelor, divorced, or widower, requires special attention and creative therapy interventions.

What value does the man place on healthy sexual functioning? What value does he place on seeing himself as being sexual as a male? How important to the man is having a good sexual and nonsexual relationship with his partner? Are there any early sexual traumas or strong religious or family prohibitions about sex that need to be addressed? How were the usual developmental tasks of adolescent sexual maturing experienced? Are there any personality factors that are contributing to the problem? (The presence of significant levels of anxiety, depression, obsessive-compulsive personality, or other neurotic or even psychotic conditions will present a challenge for treatment or even rule out the possibility for sex therapy until these problems are adequately addressed.)

The initial problem may be the complaint about erectile difficulties, but an important question is, where does the problem begin and what maintains it? Remember DAVOS?—Desire, Arousal, Vasocongestion, Orgasm, Satisfaction. Clearly failure to get or keep an erection involves vasocongestion. But which of the other modalities of DAVOS are involved in a given man's problem? Remember, there is a cascade effect between the elements of DAVOS. Therefore a difficulty in any area of the sexual response cycle can result in problems elsewhere. The end result might be erectile failure, but the questions remain. Does the unresponsive penis trace its difficulty to (1) a lack of desire; (2) failure to get or stay aroused; (3) a difficulty with orgasm or ejaculation (some men complain of loss of erection after they successfully hold back from ejaculating; others complain of "retarded ejaculation," or difficulty coming, and these same men can also experience erection loss); or (4) not being satisfied with their sexual experiences or their partner? (It is not easy to look forward to sex if you already feel that you won't enjoy it. Women know this very well, and lack of satisfaction underlies many female sexual difficulties.) Understanding where the problem may be coming from is only part of addressing a solution. The next question is how and where to intervene.

STARTING WITH PERMISSION

For many years sex therapists have used a model of therapeutic intervention that reflects different levels of need. This approach is called the PLISSIT model:

*P*ERMISSION (GIVING)
*L*IMITED *I*NFORMATION
*S*PECIFIC *S*UGGESTIONS
*I*NTENSIVE *T*HERAPY

Permission giving is a way of gleaning information from an authoritative source about what can be expected in human sexual functioning. Knowing that what you feel or the way you behave sexually is normal provides a great boost to your sexual confidence. Acquisition of knowledge alone provides an aura of permission that can help some men overcome their sexual difficulties. For example, many readers of this book will gain much insight into their sexual functioning just by learning from the description of the erection process that this book provides. For some men, such information by itself is enough to provide them with all the help they need to restore or maintain good sexual functioning. This is providing *limited information*. Many sexual concerns and difficulties can be adequately addressed by providing accurate information about sexual functioning. Men, and their partners, can take it from there.

Much of the work of sex therapy involves making *specific suggestions* that involve behavioral exercises or techniques that will reduce anxiety about sexual adequacy and enhance sexual arousal and pleasure. *Intensive therapy* might require addressing personality, relationship, and family systems issues that might be related to the sexual dysfunction. For example, some couples arrive at the sex therapist's office with complicated relationship problems in which erectile and other sexual problems are only a part of broader couple issues. In these cases, it would be useless to immediately address the sexual complaint before paying attention to the relationship itself. Couples therapy should provide or be combined with sexual therapy so that partners can learn how to foster intimacy in their relationship. Once partners achieve a comfortable level of intimacy, they can more easily move toward an increase in the level of arousal during their sexual encounters.

There are times, as mentioned in the previous paragraph, when a man who already has begun sex therapy discovers that there are underlying issues in himself or complications in his relationship that are contributing significantly to his sexual difficulties. When this happens, a shift in the focus of treatment may be necessary. It is at points such as these that it is important for the treating sex therapist to be a therapist first, who has the training and experience to recommend those interventions that may be required. The patient should expect the therapist to bring these concerns to his attention and, after discussion and agreement, perhaps make the necessary changes in the treatment plan. For example, there are times when it might be appropriate to refer a man for individual psychotherapy in order to explore and overcome resistance to sexual intimacy and the expression of emotions. This work may have to be done before "traditional sex therapy" can resume. It should be noted that the path of intensive individual therapy is not the one usually required for most men who complain of erection difficulties.

THE IMPORTANCE OF FOREPLAY

What is the role of foreplay in sexual response? For many men and their partners, foreplay is where sexual pleasure begins. The younger male with the "automatic" erection may not pay much attention to his partner during foreplay. The whole pattern of kissing, touching, and words of intimate sharing that together compose what many of us would refer to as foreplay has been called a "language" that lovers share. In a sense, foreplay is a language of communicating intimacy during which partners negotiate and share what is arousing and pleasing. Later in the book we will make suggestions about "keeping the erotic pot bubbling," which is a form of extended foreplay that for many men heightens desire.

Can foreplay itself be a part in the cause or maintenance of sexual problems? Of course it can. Foreplay is a mutual experience and sharing that for many is perhaps too intimate and, as a result, is sometimes avoided. This avoidance is especially true in long-term relationships, where the complications of daily living, along with the familiarity and predictability of the partner, can lead to a sense of sexual boredom and interpersonal discomfort.

For some men it is easier to focus on their own genital response and genital contact with their partner than to deal intimately with their partner. These men tend to bypass the variety and erotic pleasure of the language of foreplay in exchange for the conditioned eroticism of penetration and ejaculation. Feeling good is what counts! The problem is that as men age, their erections are not as "automatic." When these erections are not deemed to be "good enough" or are at times even absent, the man and his partner can be left with very little that is satisfying and intimate from their sexual encounter. It is easy to understand how the erectile problem becomes the focus of his and their sexual life.

This concern may further interfere with the intimacy of foreplay and may contribute to the ongoing problem of erectile difficulty. If a man finds himself worrying about his erections throughout foreplay, he is missing the erotic pleasure of the moment, as well as allowing performance anxiety to creep into the sexual scene. Some men are so focused on their erections that they panic if they notice some softening during prolonged foreplay. This may frequently happen, for example, while men are performing oral sex on their partner. This is not a reason for panic. This happens. The erection will return—unless it is worried away. Many men who are anxious about maintaining an erection tend to move quickly toward penetration as soon as they think they are sufficiently hard. The penis should not be rushed!

Therapists are aware that changing sexual behavior may not be as important as *changing the meaning of the behavior*. This bit of wisdom very much applies to foreplay. We are talking about a man paying attention to his partner, freely enjoying the closeness, welcoming the intimacy, and, in doing so, allowing an erection to happen and take care of itself. There is a lesson to be learned in rediscovering foreplay. Paying attention to "outercourse" and its meaning to both partners can lead to more satisfying intercourse.

There are lessons to be learned from recognizing the need to take time to focus on pleasure with one's partner as a path to sexual satisfaction, and that, while important, a good erection is only part of the sexual equation. Remember, one of the mottoes of sex therapists is that good sex is what you and your partner feel good about afterward.

A MAN NAMED BILL

The experience of a forty-seven-year-old man named Bill is a good example of how focusing on pleasure and foreplay rather than just the quality of erection can lead to a fulfilling sexual relationship. Bill was divorced and never realized just how poor the quality of sex had been in his marriage until he met Janet. She was also coming off a negative marital experience, but she was open to sex in a way that Bill had never experienced. Bill thought he was a very lucky guy to have met such a sexually responsive partner. However, he began to experience intermittent erectile problems despite really being "turned on" by Janet. The more he worried, the more inconsistent were his erections. By the time he entered treatment, he was worried as much about the failure of this new relationship as he was about the failure of his erections. He was worried that Janet would eventually reject him in bed just as his former wife would on many occasions avoid his initiations of intimacy.

With therapy, Bill soon realized that his worrying about erections only made matters worse, and that he was harming the arousal state with Janet because of thoughts of rejection and sexual frustration with his former wife. This latter insight reflects a common experience for men entering a new and important sexual relationship after years of negative sexual experience with a former partner. A man cannot be in two places (beds) at the same time! Experiencing disturbing thoughts about a former partner while trying to make love to a current partner is a recipe for failure. In Bill's case it took some time to separate the two women in his mind. Even after many successful lovemaking experiences with Janet, he still had to remain vigilant for old notions creeping back into his mind during sex. Bill learned not to let them interfere when they "bit him" without warning. He actually developed a sense of humor about them, as "old stuff" became less threatening to him. He learned not to "put his whole ego on the line" every time he and Janet had sex.

Bill gained more from therapy than just good erections. He learned about himself and his partner and developed a personal philosophy about male sexual functioning that can serve as a lesson for many men. Bill began to see himself as driven by a desire for connectedness with Janet that embraced a whole body sense of pleasure that was not limited to the genitals. He began to understand what was normal sexual functioning for him, at his age, and in his present state of life. In some instances he began to see occasional lapses from perfect erections as "normal" for him. He enjoyed his better erections but also told himself that while they might not always be as good, sex still could be good. He learned that "practice makes perfect," and tried to have an enjoyable and loving sexual experience with Janet whether or not he was "perfectly hard." He enjoyed increased self-esteem, which led to more frequent and also more enjoyable sex.

Therapists often say that even if a person has an understanding of his difficulties "in his head," that person really does not "get it" until he feels it "in his gut." In other words, an intellectual understanding of a situation or problem may not yield the same degree of change as an intuitive, experiential understanding and self-acceptance at the gut level. Bill found that his ability to reclaim his erectile capacity with Janet included both head and gut levels. But he also experienced another dimension, what he called the "heart level." Bill's breakthrough in treatment at the heart level reflected an awareness of trust and respect and absence of expectations in the relationship. For him, a lack of concern about getting an erection took the pressure off him to perform. He was not indifferent, but rather had developed an overall sense of confidence about his sexual functioning over the long run. The result was that erections were usually good, sex was regularly enjoyable to both him and his partner, and there was a greater sense of variety in their lovemaking, because it did not always have to include intercourse or even end with an orgasm. Bill learned that when it comes to sex in a committed relationship, there is always tomorrow. His sexual script had expanded as a result of treatment, thoughtful reflection, and dedicated work with a trusting and motivated partner.

INTERVENTIONS, INTERVENTIONS: AT TIMES THE PENIS NEEDS HELP

There are many men who can restore good erectile functioning by using a series of therapeutic techniques that are relatively simple. They certainly helped Bill. The difference between therapeutic success and failure often depends on commitment to work on practicing what is needed to overcome the problem. As in many aspects of life, practice makes perfect.

Many therapists agree that when it comes to dealing with a man's anxiety about sexual functioning, they are really dealing with a man's sense of self. People are validated through being accepted by a partner. Sexual failure is frequently a blow to self-validation. Both general and sexual self-image are involved in a man's experience of sexual response and "functioning." It is because of this that the targets of intervention are the reduction of anxiety and the improvement of confidence. The educational part of therapy begins with managing anxiety and enhancing desire and arousal. As confidence improves, so does self-esteem. The result is seen in better sexual functioning. What follows are some exercises that have proven to be helpful for many men.

Relaxation and imagery

Practicing simple relaxation exercises that focus on breathing, positive self-statements, and the use of positive imagery can provide a means of dealing with a host of anxiety-producing experiences, including sexual problems. The technique is simple, safe, and the person is always in control.

1. Find a quiet relaxing place. You may want to use a comfortable chair, or lie on the floor, sofa, or bed.
2. With eyes gently closed, focus on your breathing, slowly allowing day-to-day concerns to drift away as you silently say "Relax"

to yourself. Imagine life's tensions just draining away little by little with every breath you take.

3. You might want to imagine a good, comfortable, safe, and peaceful feeling filling you all over, inside and out. Go with it.

4. After a while you can silently add words like "calm" and "confident" as you repeat them over and over to yourself, allowing the meaning to sink in and a quiet inner confidence to develop.

5. Add images of how you would like to function. (Men often make the mistake of compounding their problems by imagining the worst.) Instead, imagine feeling aroused in a sexual situation and functioning the way you want to in the future.

Imagery practice should include not only anticipated positive behaviors, but also encouraging thoughts and self-statements (I am okay, this feels good, etc.), as well as feeling (pleasure, excitement, etc.). Practicing these techniques helps build confidence and reduces anxiety. Imagery practice also allows a man to check for worrisome thoughts and feelings that might arise during the imagery and may be interfering with sexual functioning. Once a man becomes aware of the negative things that he is telling himself, they can be addressed and corrected.

Practice the relaxation exercises daily and make them part of your life. Focusing on sexual functioning is an added benefit of this technique. You can imagine anything you want along the road to sexual health.

Not for beginners, but later on, once successful functioning is achieved: Do some fire drills. Men need a way of avoiding setbacks when old problems come back to "bite them" just when they thought they were okay. There may come a point when the newly restored erections "take a vacation." Practicing in imagery how one will react positively to a disappointing situation should it occur may prove to be a valuable exercise. The term "fire drill" needs no further explanation.

The stop–start technique

This has been very useful in treating both erectile and ejaculatory problems in men. Simply explained, a man is asked to masturbate until he has an erection, maintain the erection, stop the stimulation, and allow the erection to fade. After the erection has lessened or is lost, he is to start over again, masturbate until erect, and repeat the process. If he wishes, he may add a lubricant to experience a "wet sensation." Using appropriate fantasy about having good erections with his partner is also helpful. If he wishes to complete the sequence by masturbating to ejaculation, it is helpful to enjoy pairing the pleasure of orgasm with the fantasy of sex with his partner.

This same exercise can be conducted with the man's partner performing the penile stimulation. In this case, the man relaxes while his partner provides him with a pleasurable massage, then fondles him to erection, waits, allows the erection to subside, and then brings him back to erection again. If there is too much initial anxiety, then nongenital touching and holding one another is a good way to initiate contact until the man feels it is safe to move on to genital stimulation. This may take several sessions. This sequence can also be done using oral stimulation, a vibrator, and/or lubricants. Usually, the experience is pleasurable for both partners.

Stop–start practice

Many men who have erectile difficulties during intercourse are able to achieve and maintain good erections during masturbation. Despite the universality of the practice of masturbation among men (and women), there can remain a stigma for some men about self-pleasuring. Some men have been raised with religious prohibitions that fortunately are being stressed much less by various clergy today. The interplay between religion and sex will be discussed later in this book, in Chapter 24. Some men feel comfortable with solitary masturbation but would not consider it with their partners, or even want them to know about their private pleasure. (It is easy to see how this topic can become an issue for couples therapy as it speaks to whole notions about sex and relationships.) But for sex therapy and overcoming impotence, masturbation training can be a very helpful assignment. Regular masturbation is also a way of facilitating potency in men who are without partners for a length of time. There is some wisdom in the expression "Use it or lose it."

What are the benefits of the stop-start approach? Simply put, the man learns by experience that he can get an erection, and that even if it goes away, it will come back. The repetition of the exercise, alone or with the partner, reinforces the confidence that a lost erection can come back to life. For many men this knowledge alone will help greatly.

TAKING IT TO THE NEXT LEVEL

What about attempting intercourse? The best advice is again to proceed slowly. Most men are in a hurry to "try it out" right away. Sometimes their partners feel the same enthusiasm. Moving along too quickly creates the risk of experiencing renewed performance anxiety and consequent failure. Here are some hints that can help.

In the beginning, the female-on-top position for intercourse usually places less demand on the man. All he has to do initially is to lie back and enjoy the sensations of vaginal containment without worrying about his balance, placement of weight, etc. An easy way to initiate penetration is for the female partner to stimulate him to erection and to gently straddle him and place his penis in her vagina and just sit there! Let him enjoy the feeling of being hard and being inside again. This stage of on-and-off vaginal containment can be repeated, especially if he begins to lose the erection. Some gentle rocking movement by the female during containment may also help provide enough stimulation to maintain the erection. It is up to the couple to decide whether and when to move toward ejaculation. While this technique is referred to by sex therapists as "nondemand," the man still may experience some anxiety about performance. This is normal. Take the time to get comfortable. Practice makes perfect. Success builds more confidence.

There is a tendency for some men or their partners to change too quickly to other positions. Again, take time to adjust. Get used to having an erection again. Other positions may or may not work as well. Go slowly. Some positions may be more sexually arousing than others. Explore and use what works best. If there are some failures, go back to basics to regain confidence. Couples may want to go back to simple nongenital pleasuring as a way of getting to know each other again in a nonanxious and intimate sharing. This is particularly true for the future when partners may get careless and need occasionally to remember the conditions and positions that favor erections. Again, be prepared to pay some attention to the partner. Remember that doing these exercises can be both stimulating and frustrating for women. There is nothing wrong with also trying to please her while you are in the process of restoring your potency, and keep in mind that pleasing her does not require an erection. Exploring new pleasuring techniques while working on potency is a way for a couple to expand their sexual script.

Using these techniques are just some of the ways a man can help himself restore potency. There are situations when treatment may involve using a combination of medical and psychological treatments at the same time. This may include the use of mechanical aids (e.g., the vacuum pump), injection treatment, the MUSE system (a pellet introduced into the urethra), the new oral preparations (e.g., Viagra), or even surgical intervention. Again, it is important for men and their partners to be reminded that mechanical or medical intervention alone may not address personal and relationship issues that are very much a part of a man's ability to function sexually.

KEEPING UP THE GOOD WORK

Now that I can get an erection, how do I keep it? A good question. Once erectile capacity is restored, a man may be back where he started: having a sex life that is still subject to all the stresses that conspire to interfere with his enjoyment and functioning. Remember DAVOS? A man still has to pay attention to those external, internal, and interpersonal events and circumstances that either enhance or hinder his sexual functioning. Being too tired, too preoccupied, too angry at his partner, or having too much to drink, or attempting to have sex when he really isn't in the mood, are just some of the areas in which he must remain vigilant if he wants to maintain sexual health. If he encounters a new erectile problem, he should pause to understand where the problem lies: in himself, his partner, the relationship, changes in life circumstances, or something outside of current awareness. We said before that the penis doesn't lie. With this in mind, what else might be going on that is getting in the way of sexual functioning?

Maintaining sexual health is a lifelong process. There are times when successful treatment bears only temporary success. Something may have been missed during the initial treatment phase that could be returned to for further exploration, such as unresolved couple or family conflicts. This may also be time for more involved treatment in which the recurrent sexual complaints are recognized as just a symptom of deeper psychological issues. In these cases, individual or couples therapy might be necessary to explore and unlock whatever resistance underlies the sexual complaint. It must be remembered that learning from treatment failure requires actively listening to the fears and concerns of both mind and heart. This form of discernment can lead to significant growth. As we said before, sex is never simple.

13

TREATMENT FOR PHYSICAL CAUSES OF IMPOTENCE

There is perhaps no physical condition that is so humiliating, so demoralizing, and so frustrating as impotence. The ability of the penis to erect is a focus for a considerable amount of masculine self-esteem. When impotence persists for any length of time, the patient can become understandably desperate for treatment.

—Sexual Medicine Today, *June 1978*

Key Points:

- The number of options available to treat impotence that has physical causes is growing rapidly.
- Vacuum constriction devices, injections, pellets, prostheses, and oral medications are now available to treat the impotent male.
- Treatment is highly individual. Proper therapy for one patient may not be suitable for another.
- Impotence caused primarily by physical problems usually has a psychological impact, which should be addressed.

The advances made in the treatment of erectile insufficiency are nothing short of stupendous. Before exploring this exciting area, six points deserve emphasis.

1. Though relatively simple treatments are now available, *prevention is still preferable to treatment*.

2. Impotence may be the forerunner of more serious medical problems such as heart attack and stroke.

3. Impotence usually has more than one cause, and even cases that are due primarily to "physical causes" still have an impact on the psyche. Many, if not all, cases will benefit from psychological treatment and support. The National Institutes of Health notes: "Psychosocial factors are important in all forms of erectile dysfunction. Careful attention to these issues and attempts to relieve sexual anxieties should be a part of the therapeutic intervention for all patients."

4. Most often, impotence is a couples problem. Discussions between the impotent male and his partner should be encouraged, and partners should be welcomed into the doctor's or therapist's office in order to gain an understanding of the issues at hand, as well as give the partner an opportunity to lend support.

5. Impotence may be the most untreated illness in the United States for which treatment exists.

6. Erectile insufficiency exists in degrees of severity. Some cases are mild and may be transient. Some cases are progressive, while other cases are severe and possibly permanent. The appropriate treatment will depend on the cause of the erectile insufficiency as determined by the proper evaluation. Remember, the appropriate treatment for one man may not be appropriate for another.

> Knowing is not enough; we must apply.
> Willingness is not enough, we must do.
> —*Goethe*

The treatments discussed are not in order of preference. Each impotent male is an individual. The best treatment for you may differ from the best treatment for someone else.

PENILE PROSTHESES

In the 1960s and 1970s, work focused on trying to create a natural-appearing erection, and the most modern techniques involved placing a prosthesis within the phallus. The idea of having something rigid in the penis is corroborated in nature. As we noted earlier, some mammals have a bone in the penis, although humans do not. In the walrus this bone is two feet long, while in the whale it may reach thirteen feet. Among the earliest substances used to impart rigidity to the penis was a patient's own rib cartilage. But now modern science has provided us with synthetic materials.

Penile prostheses, in their modern form, were introduced in the 1960s. Improvements in design and materials led to a gradual evolution to current state-of-the-art models. There are two general types of prostheses. One (the malleable prosthesis) causes a permanent semi-rigidity in the penis, while the other (the inflatable prosthesis) allows the penis to be stiffened and relaxed depending on need. Both devices produce sufficient rigidity to allow vaginal penetration and successful intercourse.

The malleable prostheses are placed inside the erectile cylinders of the penis. They are available in different lengths and are custom-fit during a surgical procedure. These devices do not stand out at 90 degrees. They bend down when not in use and can be raised for intercourse. When the device is not in use, it is not apparent to an outside observer. A man with a prosthesis need not fear showering at the gym or fitness center in view of other males. His prosthesis will not be discernible unless the penis is grasped. If this occurs, he should probably switch exercise facilities.

The inflatable type of penile prosthesis consists of paired cylinders that fit into the erectile compartments of the penis and a fluid-containing reservoir that is placed below the skin in the lower part of the abdomen. Using a small pump that is placed inside the scrotum alongside one of the testicles, fluid may be transferred from the reservoir into the cylinders, which causes expansion, elevation of the penis, and rigidity. The inflatable prosthesis was first used in humans in 1973. Excellent results have been obtained with this device, which some have nicknamed the "erector set."

No surgical procedure is without its potential complications, and the implantation of penile prostheses is no exception. There are advantages and disadvantages to each type of device, and certain problems that are common to both. The shared problems include the possibility of infection, in which case the device will have to be removed. However, after the infection has cleared, a new prosthesis can be inserted. Another difficulty occurs if a prosthesis has been improperly fitted. If it is too long, it could cause discomfort either to the male or the female; if it is too short, it could prevent effective intercourse. However, since the devices are now available in varying widths and lengths, sizing problems are becoming less common. The device may erode through the skin, which would necessitate its removal. The prosthesis may fracture (this usually occurs during intercourse) and have to be replaced. And erectile tissue that functioned prior to insertion of the device may no longer do so.

The inflatable penile prosthesis has several advantages over the noninflatable type. It seems to give a firmer erection. Also, since the penis is extended only when the device is voluntarily inflated, it may be easier to conceal. On the other hand, there are several disadvantages to this model. There may be a mechanical failure in the pump, or the fluid inside the device may leak. The inflatable device is also more expensive and generally requires more surgical skill to implant.

The semirigid device is not perfect either. It is more likely to erode through the skin than the inflatable model, and may have to be removed. Also, some females may feel the presence of this semirigid device and may find it disturbing.

It should be apparent that with either of the above devices in place, a man is ready for action at any time. The duration of intercourse is limited only by his or his partner's fatigue.

Penile prostheses have continued to improve in their design, construction, and effectiveness. Mechanical failure of the devices is much less common than when they were first introduced. Failure rates are in the range of 10 percent in studies with between two and eight years of patient follow-up. Satisfaction surveys following implantation of penile prostheses are very impressive, with some reporting that more than 95 percent of patients are happy with the device. Interestingly, however, some patients with a functioning device discontinue use. This can be due to a change in the general health of the patient or his partner or some other factor in either of their lives.

The procedure, which used to require hospitalization, now can frequently be done on an outpatient basis. Operative time is generally between one and two hours. A patient may not use the prosthesis for intercourse until healing is complete, which usually takes between four and six weeks.

As already noted, impotence may be a serious problem for men of all ages, even older ones. Among the letters received by one urologist from patients desiring a penile prosthesis is the following:

Dear Doctor: I hope you can help me. I am ninety-two years old and recently married my second wife. She is eighty-nine years old and is a virgin. She states that she is not interested, but I truly believe she would like to have sex.

VACUUM CONSTRICTION DEVICES

Vacuum constriction devices (VCDs) were patented in 1917. Approximately seventy years passed before articles on their physiological aspects appeared in the scientific literature. VCDs are designed specifically for the penis, and the best ones require a physician's prescription.

There are many models of vacuum devices. Most are variations on the same theme and consist of a clear plastic tube into which the penis is inserted. A pump, either hand- or battery-powered, is used to create a negative pressure that draws blood into the penis. Since the plastic is clear, a male can tell when the penis is erect, and at this point a constriction type of band is placed around the base of the penis to prevent the outflow of blood. This ring should not be left in place for more than thirty minutes, since blood flow to the penis may be restricted.

A major advantage of the vacuum constriction device in that the treatment is noninvasive. Disadvantages are that some men complain of difficulty ejaculating because of the tension ring. Occasionally black-and-blue areas occur because of rupture of tiny blood vessels. These bruises gradually fade away. Some males, usually younger ones, may find the VCD cumbersome.

It is difficult to determine precisely the success rate for patients using vacuum constriction devices. However, studies have shown that after two years approximately 80 percent of men were satisfied. In addition, there was an improvement in both self-image and their relationship with their partner.

CONSTRICTION RINGS

These devices, which are placed at the base of the penis, are used primarily by those patients who have a problem with venous leakage. This condition prevents the blood from being trapped in the penis, which is necessary to produce an erection. Again, this type of device should not be left in place for more than thirty minutes.

Older males may recognize the similarity of constriction rings to "cock rings" of the past. If a male is impotent because of poor blood flow to the penis, as opposed to storage of blood within the penis, these devices are usually not helpful.

PENILE SPLINTS

While splints and supports have been in use for years, they have recently been refined. A "sleeve" fits snugly around the penis, which is then covered with a prelubricated condomlike device. The device provides sufficient support and rigidity for penetration.

Using the device is relatively risk-free. Penetration should be accomplished each time it is used. Some males or their partners find this device cumbersome, some do not.

HORMONE REPLACEMENT

Most men are aware that women who are passing through the menopause profit from the administration of hormones (estrogens). Therefore, many conclude that there must be a hormone available to resurrect a fallen phallus. Many men believe that testosterone supplementation will solve their problem of impotence.

In truth, except in extreme cases, a low-serum testosterone is more related to decreased sex drive (libido) than to erectile ability. Testosterone therapy is not usually recommended unless lab tests document low levels of the hormone.

Low levels of another hormone, dehydroepiandrosterone (DHEA), are associated with a higher likelihood of impotence. But a word of caution. It is uncertain whether taking supplements of DHEA is safe and effective in the long run. In addition, even if such supplements are helpful, proper dosages have not been determined. For now, stay away!

TOPICAL MEDICATIONS

The idea of being able to achieve an erection by applying medication to the surface of the penile skin has great appeal. Not only is it minimally invasive but it might be incorporated as part of a couple's foreplay. It is anticipated that this form of treatment would have much greater appeal than self-injections or placing a pellet in the opening of the penis. Various medications are being tested to see if an erection can be achieved in a high percentage of patients. Among those being studied are prostaglandin E2, nitroglycerin, aminophylline, and a concoction of Oriental herbs.

To date, none of these are proven therapies. More time is needed to determine their place as a treatment for impotence.

INTRAURETHRAL THERAPY

Intraurethral therapy is a relatively new way to treat erectile insufficiency. The patient inserts a small applicator, approximately one inch long, into the opening of the penis. This is done immediately after urination, which serves to lubricate the lining of the penis and facilitate insertion. Depressing a button discharges a soft pellet containing a medication called alprostadil. The male rolls his penis between his hands for ten to thirty seconds in order to dissolve and distribute the drug. Absorption into the erectile tissues occurs, and within approximately ten minutes an erection may develop, lasting from a few minutes to up to half an hour. The medication comes in various strengths, and the proper dosage must be chosen by the patient's physician.

Unlike intrapenile injections, use of which must be limited to a maximum of approximately ten times per month, the pellets may be inserted as often as every twelve hours. The device is easy to use and even blind men have mastered the technique.

Approximately 20 percent of patients will feel discomfort in the genitalia, and in a few instances blood may appear at the opening to the penis. While a prolonged erection is a possibility, it is extremely uncommon. An occasional patient will have a drop in his blood pressure, and hence the initial dose of the medicine should be given in the physician's office where pressure can be monitored.

One of the most serious potential side effects is fortunately not common. A prolonged or rigid erection lasting more than four to six hours occurs in less than 0.3 percent of patients. Most urologists who use the pellet for treating their patients have never seen such a case.

Female partners may complain of vaginal burning or itching in approximately 6 percent of cases. It is not clear whether this is due to the intraurethral pellet or merely to irritation from intercourse.

There are certain patients who should not consider using the intraurethral pellet. These include (1) patients who are known to have an allergy or adverse reaction to the active ingredient, alprostadil; (2) patients with known scarring inside the penis or penile angulation; (3) patients with sickle-cell anemia or other blood problems such as a high platelet or red blood cell count or multiple myeloma; (4) patients who have a history of thrombosis of veins; and (5) men who are having sexual intercourse with a woman who is pregnant or trying to get pregnant.

The pellets come in unopened foil packages, which should be stored in a refrigerator for maximum long-term potency. However, the pellet will remain effective for up to two weeks if left at room temperature.

A frequently asked question is whether the female is at risk when the male ejaculates, since the medication may be transferred into the vagina. To date, no ill effects have been reported, but as a precautionary measure, a couple who are trying to conceive should not use this form of therapy. No hazardous effects have been noted from oral sex (fellatio) in couples when the male is using intraurethral therapy.

It is difficult to determine the success rates of using the intraurethral pellet, but initial data indicated that 65 percent of men achieved an erection sufficient to permit intercourse. However, upon questioning, not all of these men had a rigid erection. However, "when it works it works," and these patients are generally happy.

The effectiveness of the pellet in producing an erection may be enhanced by placing a constriction ring at the base of the penis after insertion of the pellet.

The pellets are sold under the trade name MUSE, from the phrase "medicated urethral system for erections."

INTRACAVERNOUS INJECTIONS

This therapy involves the injection of medication into the erectile cylinder of the penis in order to achieve an erection that is adequate for sexual intercourse. The medication typically works within minutes, and an erection may last from several minutes to several hours.

Injection therapy was introduced into the United States at a meeting of the American Urological Association in Las Vegas in 1982. In a dramatic presentation from the podium, a British neurophysiologist, Dr. Giles Brindley, explained the procedure to his audience of physicians. He announced that a few minutes prior he had injected himself and in dramatic fashion, lowered his pants and revealed a full erection. This presentation drove home the point that an erection is caused by relaxation of the muscle in the arteries and the erectile tissue of the penis so that there is a rapid inflow of blood. The speaker following said, "I have a hard act to follow."

The FDA has approved the chemical called prostaglandin E1 (alprostadil) for use in injections. This is the same chemical used in the intraurethral therapy described earlier. Drugs for insertion are marketed under the trade names Caverject and Edex. Other effective drugs, non-FDA-approved, include papaverine and phentolamine, which may be used alone or in combination, usually with prostaglandin.

Proper dosage varies from individual to individual, and it is important that the technique be learned under the direction and supervision of a urologist. Because of the risk of scarring, which may be due to the medication and/or to the needle, it is recommended that the patient limit his use of the injections to approximately ten times per month.

Side effects of injection therapy may be divided into local and systemic reactions. The most common local reactions seen are penile pain (37 percent), prolonged erection (4 percent), scarring in the penis (3 percent), and bruising (3 percent).

It is apparent that the only common side effect is discomfort, and in the majority of cases this discomfort is rated only as mild or moderate in intensity. Less than 5 percent of patients discontinue treatment because of pain.

Systemic reactions include a rise in blood pressure (2 percent) and headache (2 percent). Thus, other than the local side effect of discomfort, there are few negative reactions.

The most serious complication is a prolonged erection, which is arbitrarily defined as one that lasts more than four hours. This complication is termed "priapism" by the medical community. It refers to an erection that persists long beyond sexual desire. The condition was named after Priapus, the Greek god of fertility. Pictures of Priapus portray him as the proud possessor of a huge, distended phallus. At first, men who develop priapism are usually pleased with their newfound prowess. However, as hours pass and the erection persists, pain develops and what was once a source of delight becomes a source of concern.

Treatment of priapism is considered an emergency. If blood remains trapped in the penis for too long, damage will occur to the erectile compartments and future erections will not be possible.

Not all men are candidates for injection therapy. Patients with an allergy to the medication, those with blood disorders such as hemophilia, sickle-cell disease, and leukemia, those with a penile implant, and those who have scarring in the penis or penile angulation are among those who should not use this form of treatment.

Some critics of the self-injection program cite a relatively high rate of discontinuation of this therapy. However, interviews with patients indicate that there are very often reasons other than lack of effectiveness that prompt them to stop. These include factors such as lack of a partner, a loss of interest in sex, or finding that they can perform with reasonable satisfaction without relying on the injection. Cost is a reason that some patients drop out but is certainly relatively low on the list. Lack of effectiveness, however, still remains a reason for discontinuation in some surveys. Interestingly, side effects of the medicine are rarely the reason that a patient stops using the injection program. The most common unfavorable reaction was discomfort. This varies greatly among patients, and most men become very comfortable with the technique and describe the discomfort of the injection as less than that of a mosquito bite. This is because the needle is so fine.

Injection therapy has had a revolutionary impact on the treatment of male sexual dysfunction. While success rates are difficult to pin down, generally 70–95 percent of men will be able to achieve satisfactory erections for intercourse. This is, in part, dependent on which medications are used. Partner satisfaction rates are generally around 60–70 percent.

The self-injections have been approved as treatment for impotence with either physical or psychological causes.

SURGERY FOR PROBLEMS OF BLOOD FLOW TO THE PENIS

Erection in the male is dependent upon two major factors: adequate inflow of blood into the erectile cylinders, and containment of blood within those cylinders. As has been noted, there is no bone in the human penis as exists in other mammals such as the whale, walrus, and dog.

Surgical success in bringing more blood flow to the heart is well documented in both the medical and lay communities. This procedure, known as coronary artery bypass grafting and cardiac revascularization, has become one of the most commonly performed procedures in the United States. The outstanding success rate raises the question of whether a similar procedure could be developed for bringing more blood to the impaired penis in impotent males. A number of physicians have devoted a great amount of time and effort to try to make this a reality. Multiple surgical techniques have been outlined in medical literature. As is usually the case when as many as a half-dozen surgical techniques are described, no one method has proved to be highly successful. Such is the case with penile revascularization. Success rates in follow-up studies have been disappointing, and at this time it is a procedure that is applicable for only a limited number of patients and should be performed only by a urologist who has extensive experience in this area.

While most operations designed to increase blood flow to the penis have mixed results, there is one circumstance in which the procedure does well. It is usually seen in younger men who have a history of difficulty obtaining erections after some form of trauma to the pelvis. Examples are injuries from an automobile accident, a fall, or a bicycle accident. In these cases surgery is performed on a relatively large blood vessel that has a short area of blockage. Relieving this blockage increases the blood flow to the smaller vessels of the penis that are responsible for erection. This is not to be confused with the surgical treatment of impotence caused by decreased blood flow to the penis from narrowing of the smaller blood vessels. In these instances, it is much more difficult to restore blood flow.

Very recent studies indicate that it may be possible to induce the regeneration of blood vessels in the heart through use of certain medication. One may speculate that if this proves successful, a similar technique may be helpful in correcting the problem of impaired blood flow to the penis.

SURGERY FOR PROBLEMS OF STORAGE OF BLOOD IN THE ERECTION COMPARTMENTS

Even if the flow of blood to the erectile cylinders of the penis is adequate, there is another vascular problem that may prevent a successful erection. This is called "venous leak." Recall that a successful erection depends upon expansion of the erectile tissue within the penis to the extent that the normal drainage channels (the emissary veins) are compressed against the firm lining of the erectile cylinders. If the compression mechanism does not function properly, then the blood that should accumulate is allowed to escape and no erection occurs. Some specialists believe that this may be a more common problem than impaired blood flow into the erectile cylinders.

As is the case with surgery designed to bring more blood to the penis, multiple operations have been described to correct the problem of venous leak. Unfortunately, follow-up data collected two years after the procedure have been disappointing, with less than a 50 percent success rate. It may help a properly selected number of patients but should be performed only by urologists who specialize in this area.

14

A NEW ERA BEGINS:
INTRODUCTION OF VIAGRA AS THE FIRST ORAL AGENT TO TREAT IMPOTENCE

Luck is where preparation meets opportunity.

—*Author unknown*

Key Points:

- The first oral medication to treat impotence has been approved by the FDA.
- Sildenafil citrate (Viagra) is highly effective in treating men with impotence.
- The medication works in most men whether the cause is physical or psychological.
- The drug is remarkably well tolerated, with very few side effects.
- Any male taking medication containing nitrates should not use sildenafil.
- While the medication is approved only for use in males, it is quite likely it will treat "female impotence."

March 27, 1998, was a historic day in the field of impotence. The FDA granted clearance for use of the first oral agent to treat male erectile insufficiency. Sildenafil citrate, manufactured by Pfizer Labs, is distributed under the trade name Viagra. Viagra, a blue tablet, comes in three strengths: 25, 50, and 100 milligrams. The clinical studies leading to the FDA's approval of Viagra can be briefly summarized. In twenty-one studies, Viagra was administered to more than three thousand patients ranging in age from nineteen to eighty-seven years. The average male had been impotent for five years. Men taking Viagra demonstrated significant improvement in erections in all studies. Viagra was effective in helping males both to attain and to sustain an erection. The degree of effectiveness was related to the dose. Approximately 63 percent of males responded to a 25 mg dose, 74 percent to a 50 mg dose, and 82 percent to a 100 mg dose. The usual starting dose is 50 mg. If a male does not succeed at this level, then 100 mg should be tried at the next sexual encounter. On the other hand, if 50 mg is successful, it is recommended to reduce the dose to 25 mg.

There are times when a physician may change the starting dose of Viagra for his patient. For example, men over sixty-five years old eliminate the medication more slowly from the bloodstream than younger males and may require a lower dose. In addition, patients who have significant kidney or liver disease should use a reduced dosage. This is a decision for your physician.

The use of certain other drugs may also require dosage adjustment. For example, patients who are taking cimetidine (Tagamet), erythromycin, ketoconazole, or itraconazole will have higher blood levels of Viagra in their bloodstream after taking a pill than patients who are not on these types of medicines. This is due to the fact that these medicines may interfere with the metabolism of the medication. In these instances, Viagra is generally safe to use but at a lower dose.

Viagra works in a unique way. It blocks the enzyme (phosphodiesterase type 5) that is responsible for destroying the chemical (cyclic guanosine monophosphate) that causes relaxation of the erectile tissue in the penis and allows the inflow of blood necessary to produce an erection. (See Chapter 4, "Understanding Erections.") After swallowing, Viagra is readily absorbed and reaches its highest level in the bloodstream in approximately one to two hours. However, many patients have noticed that taking Viagra one and a half to two hours before sexual activity produces better results. A high-fat meal may delay the absorption and the onset of action of the medication. For example, if a man eats fettucini Alfredo for dinner and takes the pill with his meal, he needs to allow for the fact that the medication will take longer to be absorbed and reach its maximum effectiveness.

The statement "it's too good to be true" does not apply to Viagra. It is good and it is true. The drug is highly effective, yet has remarkably few side effects. Those reported, along with frequency of occurrence, in studies submitted to the FDA included:

Headache—16%
Flushing—10%
Indigestion—7%
Nasal congestion—4%
Urinary tract infection—3%
Increased light sensitivity/blurred vision or colored tinge—3%
Diarrhea—3%
Dizziness—2%
Rash—2%

It should be noted that all of these side effects were generally mild and rarely did a patient have to stop the drug. Viagra has not been shown to produce cancer or impair fertility.

Although Viagra is generally safe, there is one *absolute* reason not to use it. Any patient who is taking medication containing nitrates in any form should not take Viagra, as it may cause a significant and serious drop in blood pressure. Depending upon circumstances, it is possible that a heart attack or stroke could occur.

Following the introduction of Viagra, there were a limited number of deaths associated with its use. The actual number was relatively small when compared to the total number of patients using the drug. Many of these deaths were thought to be due to a heart attack. In some cases it occurred in patients who were already using medications containing nitrates. This is the one circumstance in which a patient should never use Viagra. There are no exceptions. Some deaths occurred in patients who were not using nitrates, and it is believed that a heart attack or abnormal rhythm of the heart was precipitated by the physical demands of sexual intercourse.

Clearly, there is a degree of cardiac risk associated with sexual activity, although in fact it is relatively low. (See Chapter 20.) Physicians and patients need to take into account whether or not there is a history of heart problems before initiating treatment. The American College of Cardiology in conjunction with the American Heart Association has recommended caution in prescribing Viagra for patients with certain medical profiles. These include:

1. Patients with active coronary artery disease
2. Patients with a history of congestive heart failure and borderline low blood pressure
3. Patients who are already taking multiple drugs for high blood pressure
4. Patients who are on drugs such as erythromycin or cimetidine or have conditions such as liver or kidney disease that can prolong the amount of Viagra in the circulation

Sexual activity does impose some increased stress and demands on the heart. If a patient has taken Viagra and develops chest pain from sexual activity and is taken to the emergency room, he must inform the physician that he has used the medication. It would not be uncommon to administer medication containing nitrates to such a patient, and the combination could be dangerous. This should not frighten those who are appropriate candidates to use Viagra or keep them from using the medicine. The fact is that most patients, even those with a previous history of cardiac problems, will not develop chest pain during sexual activity.

The overwhelming majority of patients can safely use this miracle medication. How many tablets should be taken in a twenty-four-hour period? It is recommended that no more than one tablet be used every twenty-four hours. And Viagra should not be used in combination with any other form of treatment for impotence, such as the intraurethral pellet or self-injections. This is an area that has not been adequately studied, so caution is advised.

Despite the fact that the drug is remarkably safe, it still should be used only with a physician's advice. In addition, it should be emphasized, as Pfizer Labs has done, that "a thorough medical history and physical examination should be undertaken to diagnose erectile dysfunction, determine potential underlying causes and identify appropriate treatment." In simple terms, a man should not use this medication until he has been properly assessed by a physician. Hence, this medication, like all prescription medications, should never be borrowed or shared with a friend.

QUESTIONS COMMONLY ASKED ABOUT VIAGRA

1. Will Viagra increase sex drive?

Viagra is not an aphrodisiac per se. However, many impotent males who find that they can perform using Viagra do feel invigorated. It is not unusual for them to have a heightened interest in sexual activity, and this may result in increased frequency of intercourse. Men who have enjoyed a restoration of their potency because of Viagra often are giddy about their newfound prowess.

2. Will Viagra treat premature ejaculation?

Viagra is not a standard treatment for premature ejaculation. Most men with premature ejaculation generally do not have any problem maintaining an erection until they ejaculate. It simply happens too soon. Viagra will not prolong the time between erection and ejaculation. However, if a male is losing his erection prior to ejaculation, then it may be very helpful. Also, Viagra may help by decreasing the time to attain the next erection.

3. Will Viagra help the non-impotent male?

Viagra should not improve erectile ability in a normal male. This is because a man who is having no problem with impotence already has enough of the chemical (nitric oxide) that causes an erection available, and adding more simply will not help. It is much like continuing to fill an already full gas tank.

4. Will Viagra increase orgasmic intensity?

From a strictly physiological standpoint, one would not expect Viagra to increase the intensity of orgasm. However, many men report that it does. This may be because males who could not perform prior to using Viagra are now experiencing a pleasurable sensation for the first time in many years. In addition, because orgasm is a mind-body phenomenon, the sensation of orgasm may be heightened psychologically.

5. Will Viagra decrease the time it takes to achieve successive erections?

Following ejaculation there is an amount of time called the "refractory period" before a male can achieve his next erection. Many men taking Viagra report that they are able to achieve a subsequent erection following ejaculation sooner than usual. For them this is an unexpected and welcome bonus.

6. Will Viagra "prevent impotence"?

The answer to this question is unknown, but there is a scientific and intuitive reason to believe that it might help. In the erect state, blood that is rich in oxygen helps keep the erectile tissue of the penis healthy. Many patients taking Viagra report that they experience nocturnal and morning erections that they have not had for years. It is therefore possible that with an increase in these erections the erectile tissue of the penis will remain healthy, since it receives more oxygen-rich blood. It is known that erectile tissue that does not receive oxygen-rich blood tends to form scar, which inhibits erectile ability. These findings beg the question as to whether one day men will take oral medication to prevent impotence. This thinking has not yet been proved in scientific studies and is speculative. At this time Viagra is not approved by the FDA as a preventive medication for impotence.

7. Will Viagra help women?

A logical question is whether Viagra will help women with sexual problems. Studies are underway in this regard. Since there are similarities between erectile tissue in men and women and since Viagra has been shown to increase blood flow to female organs such as the clitoris and vagina, it holds great promise.

For many years, women's sexual problems have been thought to be primarily psychological in origin, "in their heads," and have been largely ignored. The success of Viagra has caused a flood of interest from the pharmaceutical industry, which is hoping to capture the women's market. What are the sexual problems that most women experience and that the pharmaceutical industry hopes to address? They include lack of interest in sex, inability to achieve orgasm, problems with arousal and vaginal lubrication, and an overall lack of pleasure from sexual activity. Some women have already taken Viagra and feel it helps, but appropriate studies must be conducted before the answer is known.

THE FUTURE

Now that researchers better understand how an erection occurs, other medications are in development to treat male impotence. These include phentolamine and apromorphine. These drugs are chemically different from Viagra, as well as from each other. In addition, a topical cream containing alprostadil is being developed. We can expect other medications to become available in future years.

An intriguing relationship between certain scents and sexual arousal is beginning to be explored. Research in this area may pave the way for finding new ways to increase libido and manage sexual problems.

The importance of scent has long been recognized in animals. Mating cycles revolve around the release of chemicals called pheromones. But in humans the effect of scent on sexuality is as yet undefined. It is known, however, that tissue not only in the genitalia but also in the nose becomes engorged during periods of sexual stimulation.

Certain scents are known to increase sexual arousal. In men, genital blood flow has been demonstrated to increase in reaction to the following aromas or combinations of scents. The number in parenthesis represents the average increase in blood flow to the genitalia:

Lavender and pumpkin pie	(40%)
Licorice and doughnuts	(32%)
Pumpkin pie and doughnuts	(20%)
Cinnamon buns	(4%)

In women, sexual arousal, as measured by increased blood flow, is enhanced by the following scents:

Good & Plenty candy and cucumber	(13%)
Baby powder	(13%)

Good & Plenty candy and banana nut bread   (12%)
Lavender and pumpkin pie   (11%)
Baby powder and chocolate   (4%)
Women's perfume   (1%)

Certain odors may "turn off" a female's interest in sexual activity. In women, sexual arousal is decreased by the scent of cherry and charcoal barbecue smoke. No turn-offs were found in men.

We are a long way from a complete scientific understanding of the effects scents have on human sexual arousal. However, continued research may point the way to new forms of treatment for certain sexual problems or enhanced sexual pleasure. Who knows what the future holds? Will we one day use nasal sprays in order to get aroused? Will there be specially scented birthday and anniversary cards or stationery?

15

RESTORING ERECTIONS MAY NOT SOLVE RELATIONSHIP PROBLEMS

The reason so many women fake orgasm is that so many men fake foreplay.

—*Terry Tafoya, Ph.D.*

Key Points:

- The introduction of new oral agents to treat impotence will be greatly welcomed by many men and their partners.
- Relationship problems may still get in the way of satisfactory sex despite the restoration of the ability to have erections.
- There are psychological responses by both partners to the return of erectile capacity.

The introduction of Viagra for the treatment of erectile failure and the promise of a future generation of specific medical interventions give great hope of a return to sexual health for many men and their partners. The latest treatment choices are added to the existing interventions, which include transurethral pellets (e.g., MUSE), injection treatment (e.g., Caverject and Edex), vacuum pumps, penile prostheses, and traditional sex therapy techniques. Each of these treatments has been successful in restoring some men's capacity to have erections. The recent introduction of Viagra has brought dramatic attention to the ease of restoring erections through the use of a specific medication. What can men and their partners expect now that a new era of the treatment of erectile failure has been made possible with the introduction of such new methods of treating impotence? A whole host of questions are answered while other issues are raised when erection problems are "cured" through the tools of modern medicine.

For many men and their partners, existing medical treatment such as Viagra and others in the process of development will provide just what they were seeking: good, reliable erections that will make their episodes of impotence and erectile difficulties a past memory. These men will be able to resume an active sex life free of old worries about erectile failure, whether their problems came from physical or psychological causes or a combination. Even men who did not have significant erectile difficulties may find a boost of confidence and performance from this medication to the point that their overall interest in sex will be enhanced. For many men, performance anxiety will be a thing of the past. If there is spectatoring, it will be to enjoy the quality of the erections and pleasure rather than to worry about adequate performance. These men and their partners will be grateful for this major advance in sexual medicine. Thanks to new medication, their overall levels of sexual desire and arousal may increase, and there may be a general improvement in sexual and marital satisfaction. Many couples may even "live happily ever after."

PSYCHOLOGICAL ISSUES ONCE ERECTIONS ARE RESTORED

The return to sexual health creates a psychological response and adjustment to the positive outcome of treatment. A truly positive outcome may require more than just being able to have reliable erections. For many men and their partners, no matter how effective the medication and no matter how great the promise of reliable medically assisted erections, there may still be some unanswered questions about their sexual relationships. Once the ability to have erections is restored, new issues for the man and his partner might be raised. Many of the relationships issues addressed elsewhere in this book will still be important in determining the ongoing quality of their common sexual life. The psychological causes of impotence outlined in Chapter 5, such as personal development, the couple's sexual script, and the capacity for intimacy, will still play a part in how a couple respond to the capacity to have reliable erections. They may even find themselves facing sexual problems similar to those couples who never had erection problems but still had personal or relationship-based sexual difficulties.

Let us list a few of the difficulties for a man or his partner that might exist after potency has been restored. Were there problems relating for the partners before the advent of using Viagra or other treatment agents? Some men may find that they do not use the medication even if they have it. There are men who do not even get the prescription filled! What is going on here? Perhaps such a man really does not want help! It is worth exploring.

A man may be ambivalent about his motivation to "cure" his erection problem. Perhaps a return to sexual functioning might not solve the "real" problem and may even create new ones. For example, his partner may be nonorgasmic, or perhaps sexually repressed, and a return to potency might lead him to further sexual frustration with her. By maintaining his impotence, the man retains an intact equilibrium with his partner in what might otherwise be a satisfying relationship. She may even find comfort in his impotence, knowing he will not act out sexually with other women. In fact, he may be using his impotence in the same way—as a safeguard of his fidelity to his partner. The status quo is thus maintained by the male's not taking advantage of a "cure" for his impotence. For another couple, the dynamic might differ in that the functional partner may have an investment in the dysfunctional partner remaining that way. This status will provide an excuse to seek other partners while still enjoying the benefits of a comfortable relationship.

Other questions come to mind that can have a bearing on a man and his partner's response to the restoration of the sexual functioning. For example, did the couple adequately discuss and resolve the problems that led to the original complaints of impotence? Now that the potential for reliable erections has been restored, have they addressed the lifestyle, relationship, and sexual script issues that may have originally contributed to and could still be maintaining the present problems? The same "turn-ons" and "turn-offs" about sex could still be present, regardless of the availability or use of medication. Remember, even with the restored capacity for erections, not all "successful" sex is "satisfying" sex. A chemically assisted erection may not result in either increased sexual desire or a subjective state of arousal.

From the man's perspective, his newfound potency can have an enormous impact on his sense of self. On the one hand, he may feel great about being able to function effectively, while on the other hand he may feel that he may be called upon to have "sex on demand." He is not as important as his erections. No excuses, just take the pill! Of course, his partner may feel the same pressure to be always available for him. We have already discussed that if he was not really attracted to his partner, his erectile difficulties could have been a sign of that dissatisfaction. The same experience could have been true for his partner, who may have been relieved that he was impotent. It could be that because of new medical advances both partners are now left without an excuse to avoid sexual intimacy. Now that they have the chance to be intimate, they may actually be out of practice or not even interested. There is also the possibility that previously undiscovered relationship and sexual problems in either partner will be uncovered as a result of the restoration of potency. Some couples will benefit from some counseling to help them face the potential effects of change in potency on their sexual relationship. Many factors could be at work, and, as mentioned elsewhere in this book, the issues of power, trust, and intimacy continue to be underlying agents in any sexual relationship.

From a partner's perspective, the medically assisted return of potency for the male can of course be met with positive relief. On the other hand, a woman may feel the pressure that sex will now be "on demand" and will not take her readiness into account. The notion of her partner "taking a pill" may go against her idea of sex as a spontaneous event for partners. Yet other women would be quite willing to exchange spontaneity of sex for dependability of their partner's erections. She may no longer be able to use his erections as a sign that she turns him on. A woman may even be angry or resentful that the man is getting over his erectile problem without having to pay attention to the quality of their relationship. Again, she may have not cared much for sex in the first place and preferred him to be impotent. These and other problems may reflect the general state of the partner relationship, and such concerns should be addressed. We can see that in some cases a guaranteed erection may not be a guarantee of a pleased partner.

A man's restoration to potency may also result in a change in the dynamics of the couple. A partner may feel that the man is not as dependent on her as he once was when he had erectile difficulties. Will she become less important in his eyes? She may be concerned about his health now that sexual activity can be resumed. (Of course, health concerns by either partner about taking medication and resuming sexual activity should be discussed with the treating physician.) She may even feel threatened and insecure about issues of fidelity. It is true that some men will try out their restored potency with new partners. Even if this is a passing activity, it can still create a significant problem for the couple.

The restoration of potency may understandably tempt the couples once again to focus exclusively on intercourse. They may be in a hurry to begin penetration and not take their time in preparation for lovemaking. Depending on the level of their customary attentiveness to sexual expression before the medication became available, the couple might be reminded to focus on foreplay. They also need to pay attention to how they negotiate the when, where, and how of their sexual activity. Again, there is a need for partners to be reminded that more is involved in obtaining sexual satisfaction than just having an adequate erection.

Overall, it appears that the advent of medications such as Viagra and other treatments that restore erectile functioning will be of enormous benefit to many men and their partners. For some, this medical intervention will be all they need to restore a satisfying sex life. It will enable them to talk more openly about sex and improve their overall enjoyment. Other men, especially those whose original erectile difficulties were related to psychological or a combination of physical and psychological causes, may use their restoration of potency as a sufficient reason not to explore the psychological and relationship components of their problem. Sadly, an opportunity for further growth will be lost.

As we have seen, the benefits of the restoration of sexual functioning always occur within the context of an individual man and his relationships. Even the positive experience of moving from sexual malfunction to healthy sexual functioning will bring about a ripple effect of changes in the interactions of a man and his partner. Depending on the couple, even such positive changes toward sexual health may benefit from support and professional guidance as a couple reclaims the potency and intimacy that had been lost. Those couples for whom the restoration of potency does not solve their relationship problems or causes them to become aware of new issues in their sexual lives can also benefit from taking the time to explore these issues with a trained professional. When it comes to satisfaction in matters of relating sexually, time will tell. If counseling is needed, people eventually know something needs to be done.

16

A WORD OF CAUTION:
WHAT *NOT* TO DO

The progress of rivers to the sea is not as rapid as
that of man to error.

—Voltaire

Key Points:

Will any of the following solve the problem of impotence?

"Magic medicine" and "quick cures"
A visit to a prostitute
Treatment at a "massage" parlor
"Spanish fly"
Homemade penile rings
Withholding sex
Pornography
Borrowed medication

The answer is "No!"

It takes a certain amount of frustration and courage for a male to
decide to seek help for erectile insufficiency. Many individuals are reluctant to visit a doctor, either because they are embarrassed or because
they do not know how to bring up the problem. Many may seek a
"quick cure." Most such cures are a waste of time, money, and effort.

"MAGIC MEDICINE" AND "QUICK CURES"

Pornographic magazines advertise a dazzling array of medicines and devices that are supposed to solve such problems as erectile failure and premature ejaculation. Other products are designed for the male who is unable to bring his female partner to orgasm. Creams and lotions are advertised that supposedly allow a male to "get it up again and again and again." "Hard-on" pills, as well as recipes that combine such aphrodisiacs as sarsaparilla and kola nut, are touted as promoting sexual potency on command. The various devices available boggle the mind. "Cock rings" are stated to provide a rock-hard erection. Battery-powered rubber vibrating devices that fit around the penis promise to produce an erection. A vibrating plug that is inserted into the male's rectum is supposed to provide a sensation that causes an immediate erection.

For men who are having difficulty with a live partner, there are life-sized dolls with various-sized vaginas. These dolls can be placed in several positions. Some are even battery-powered and have a vibrating device built into the vagina or rectum. One of the more intriguing models even talks and moans in simulated ecstasy. Stores sell innumerable gadgets that could help an impotent man stimulate his partner. Vibrators, clitoral stimulators, and dildos come in various sizes and shapes.

None of the above items has been scientifically proved to solve the problem of impotence, but it would be shocking to calculate the millions of dollars spent on such devices by frustrated, desperate men who know of no other way to find help.

Also, one must be wary of bold headlines in the press. While most newspapers and magazines have a well-trained, professional staff, not all do. A classic example occurred in an article that initially appeared in *Scientific American*. The work of Beverly Whipple and Barry Komisaruk on female sexuality was accurately featured. The *Times* of London did a spoof suggesting that the researchers were on the verge of discovering an "orgasm pill." This was picked up by the *New Brunswick Home News & Tribune*. Information was twisted so that the reader was led to believe that a pill for orgasm was forthcoming. Other publications then picked up the erroneous message with titillating headlines such as "Orgasm Pill

Is Close to Climax" (*The People of London*). The *New York Post* stated dramatically, "Thrill Pill for Women Could Be Here Soon." The *Evening Standard* drew attention with the headline, "Sex Pill Cuts Out the Middle Man." None of these headlines reflected the true content of the initial article. So, be a healthy skeptic when it comes to dramatic headlines.

WILL A PROSTITUTE HELP?

Nearly every man who is impotent has wondered at some time whether he might be able to have an erection and successful intercourse with a new partner. And some men feel that a very experienced female, such as a prostitute, might be able to stimulate them sufficiently to enable them to perform. These individuals suppose that a prostitute knows certain techniques that would ensure a good erection.

However, most men who are impotent will not derive any benefit from a prostitute. Men who have primarily a physical cause for their impotence will not benefit from the dreamed-of sexual stimulation provided by a prostitute. And men who are impotent for psychological reasons are no more likely to benefit, since what they most often need is a sympathetic and understanding female partner. Obviously, most prostitutes do not meet this need. Patient foreplay, which an impotent male very much needs, usually does not take place during a sexual encounter with a prostitute. Furthermore, the very knowledge that a man is dealing with a professional may create self-imposed demands that he cannot fulfill. The male will be more concerned with performance than with enjoyment and almost certainly will not be able to achieve an erection because of anxiety.

A less threatening environment may be a "massage parlor." Such establishments exist in virtually every major city in the United States. However, few men know what will occur when they go for a "massage." While differences between massage parlors do exist, most treatments consist of a general body massage, culminating in a "local," which consists of a genital massage, usually lasting no more than a few minutes.

An interesting survey characterized the patrons of massage parlors. The typical customer is white, thirty-five years old, and married. He has had at least thirteen years of education and is employed in a lower- or middle-class occupation. He is a regular churchgoer. He has probably come to the massage parlor because he is dissatisfied with his sexual partner, unable to perform, or simply curious. Personality evaluation reveals that these men generally have high self-esteem and consider themselves personally and sexually well adjusted.

When queried as to whether they came for the massage or the "local," 40 percent of the men interviewed stated that they came for the massage, 40 percent for the "local," and 20 percent for both. But 35 percent of the patients failed to reach orgasm during the genital massage.

In short, for men who are having difficulties, a massage parlor is a poor place to try to work out the problem. The atmosphere itself is anxiety-producing and the genital massage is strictly mechanical. There is no time for the emotional support or encouragement that the impotent male needs.

"SPANISH FLY"

Many men believe this may be the "wonder drug" for curing impotence. Over the years, great claims have been made for the drug's ability to arouse a man or woman.

The famous French surgeon Ambroise Paré wrote an interesting account of an overdose of Spanish fly:

> In 1572, we went to see a poor Argonian man in Provence, who was affected by the most horrible and frightful satyriasis one could ever see. The fact is: he had Quartan fever. To cure it, he consulted an old sorceress who made him a potent composed of an ounce and a half of nettles and two drams of Cantharides which made him so hardened in the venereal act that his wife swore to us by her god that he had been astride her during two nights, 87 times, without thinking it more than ten . . . and even while we were interviewing him, the poor man ejaculated thrice in our presence.

The active ingredient in Spanish fly is cantharidin. The Spanish fly is in fact a beetle, found in central and southern Europe, which is dried and then powdered. It is an extremely irritating substance, and when taken internally it may indirectly cause an erection. However, serious side effects of cantharidin include severe abdominal pain, frequent and painful urination, and even the passage of some bits of tissue that come from inside the irritated penis. It can be a very dangerous drug and should not be tried.

MECHANICAL DEVICES

One should not insert any object into the opening of the penis in order to stiffen it. Such objects can become lodged so that they require surgical removal. An object sometimes inserted inside the penis is a swizzle stick used to mix cocktail drinks. This object may be commonly chosen because it is convenient, particularly if a man has had several drinks and has a great desire for sex but fears his performance will be inadequate.

Also, one should not put any type of ring around the penis to make it stiff. Swelling generally occurs, and the ring cannot be removed. In many instances, surgery is necessary to relieve the predicament. One young male placed a solid metal ring at the base of his penis; several hours later, he found it could not be removed. It was like a ring stuck on a finger. In the emergency room all the known tricks, including using soap and water and Vaseline, were attempted. The patient was taken to the operating room and anesthetized, but further attempts at removal were unsuccessful. The ring was made of cast iron, and no instrument available in the operating room could even scratch its surface. A consultation was then held with a plumber who happened to be on late duty at the hospital. The plumber changed from his usual clothes into a surgical scrub suit and entered the operating room. After examining the patient, he said, "You'll have to cut it off." When asked what instrument could be used to cut off the ring, he responded, "Nothing will cut that ring; you'll have to cut off the penis." However, the penis was preserved by cutting off all its outer skin, which permitted the ring to slide off. The skin was then grafted back into place.

In an attempt to prolong an erection, some men or their female partners have applied a rubber band or tied a string to the base of the penis, the idea being to block the drainage of blood from the penis and thus keep it erect. However, this is extremely dangerous and may result in gangrene of the organ. Constriction rings specifically designed and manufactured for the penis are a much better choice (see Chapter 13).

WITHHOLDING SEX

Some men who have difficulty achieving erections feel that they would perform better if their female partner were more sexually aggressive. Some men actually fantasize being attacked, or virtually raped, by their female partner. Many men would find that if they openly discussed this desire with their partner, the latter would willingly cooperate. However, most males are too embarrassed to bring up the subject. A man may then decide that if he withholds sex from his female partner, she will become ravenous for sex and thus fulfill all of his wishes. This ploy seldom works. The male finds himself becoming increasingly frustrated sexually as his desire for intercourse increases, and all the while, he is still uncertain whether he will be able to achieve an erection when the times comes. Meanwhile, his partner may not seem to notice that a significant amount of time has elapsed since the last sexual act, and this becomes of great concern to the male, who now wonders if she really ever wants to have sexual relations again. On the other hand, the female may be very aware of the sudden cessation of sexual activity, and she may erroneously conclude that her partner is no longer interested in sex. Thus, both parties draw the wrong conclusions and neither benefits.

WILL PORNOGRAPHY HELP?

Some men who are having difficulty getting an erection wonder whether they might be successful if they were stimulated by pornographic material. Today, there is an abundance of such matter available either in the form of "adult movies" or very explicit magazines. There is no doubt that different men are stimulated by different types of subject matter. Thus, one finds movies or books dealing not only with heterosexual activity but also with lesbianism, group orgies, anal intercourse, and "discipline," in which women are subjected to various types of sadistic treatment. In 1976 approximately one hundred such films were produced. Twenty years later the number had risen to eight thousand. Many video rental stores report that "adult films" are their biggest moneymakers.

Many impotent men have purchased either movies or magazines and have viewed them at home while attempting to masturbate or even while trying to engage in intercourse. Some have even devised a rather elaborate setup that permits the movie to be shown on the ceiling above the bed. There is no doubt that males who are not having difficulties may be readily stimulated by this material and will quickly develop a hard erection. But most men who are impotent do not find that this alleviates their problem, because it does not address the underlying physical and/or psychological problems. Despite the fact that they may find this material sexually arousing, they still can't get an erection.

BORROWED MEDICINE

Never, never use medicine that has not been prescribed specifically for you. As problems with impotence become more openly discussed, men are more likely to learn that a friend may have received some type of medication for treating impotence from a physician. Some impotent men will reason, "If it works for him it will work for me." This is extremely dangerous reasoning. Some medicines may have undesirable side effects on certain individuals and not on others. In addition, you may be taking another medication that your friend is not and that will cause a serious drug interaction.

Recently in an emergency room, a urologist received a phone call from the emergency room physician at three o'clock on Saturday morning. A sixty-year-old male had come in with priapism (a sustained erection that will not go away). As the story unraveled, it was learned that the patient had borrowed a friend's medication for penile self-injection and given himself a shot. A prolonged erection occurred, which ultimately become painful and required drainage of blood from the penis in the emergency room.

TOPICS OF
SPECIAL INTEREST

17

SEXUAL PERFORMANCE AND AGING

To know how to grow old is a master work of
wisdom, and one of the most difficult chapters in
the great art of living.

—Frederic Amiel

Key Points:

- Impotence is not inevitable in older males.
- Impotence is not caused by aging but is associated with other illnesses.
- Significant physiological changes do normally occur in a male's sexual ability as he ages, but impotence is not one of them if he is otherwise healthy.
- The older male may be better able to satisfy his female partner than the younger male.
- Society should not regard older males who retain their interest in sex as "dirty old men."

As life expectancy in the United States increases, more and more "senior citizens" and their partners have questions regarding sexual issues. This trend is expected to continue.

At the turn of the century (1900), only approximately 4 percent of the United States population was older than sixty-five years. By the turn of the next century (2000), it is expected that at least 20 percent of the population will be over sixty-five.

At age sixty-five, the average male may expect to live another seventeen or eighteen years. At age seventy-five, twelve years of additional life is average, and by age eighty-five, the average male may expect to live an additional seven years. In the older male, the level of sexual activity is governed to some degree by whether or not he has a partner and the general health of that individual.

In older males, sexual activity may be of less importance. The decline in importance may be independent of the individual's general health. However, it is clear that individuals who are in generally good health are more likely to have sexual activity.

NORMAL CHANGES IN SEXUAL FUNCTION WITH AGING

There are so many preconceived notions about aging that many men feel impotence is simply an inevitable part of growing older. The truth is that erectile insufficiency is *not* caused by aging. It is a phenomenon that occurs with the onset of other illnesses, and since the likelihood of illness increases with age, so does impotence.

As males grow older, certain alterations in sexual functioning do occur. These include the following:

1. It takes longer to achieve an erection.
2. The duration of ejaculation decreases from between four and eight seconds to approximately three seconds.
3. The volume of the ejaculate is reduced from approximately one teaspoon to less than half that amount.
4. The force with which the semen is expelled decreases so that it is projected from the end of the penis a distance of only two to twelve inches instead of twelve to twenty-four inches.
5. The time from erection to ejaculation may be increased.
6. Following ejaculation the penis becomes soft much more rapidly.
7. The time before the next erection can be achieved is prolonged.
8. The weight of the testicles decreases.
9. The tactile sensitivity of the penis decreases.

10. The intensity of the orgasm may decrease.
11. The upward angle of erection also decreases.

The above are *normal* changes that occur as the years pass, but note that erectile insufficiency is *not* a part of the aging process. Erectile ability is in fact associated with a male's general health status. Men in their eighties who are otherwise healthy will be able to have erections. Thus, maintaining good general health is a key to preventing impotence.

ERECTILE ABILITY IN EACH DECADE

Sexual activity by decade has been humorously depicted:

> 20–30 years: Tri-daily
> 30–40 years: Tri-weekly
> 40–50 years: Try-weakly
> 50–60 years: Try-oysters
> 60–70 years: Try anything
> 70–80 years: Try to remember

It has also been described more poetically:

> *From 20 to 30,*
> *If a man lives right,*
> *It's once in the morning*
> *And once at night.*

> *From 30 to 40,*
> *If a man lives right,*
> *It's once in the morning*
> *But seldom at night.*

> *From 40 to 50*
> *It's now and then;*
> *From 50 to 60*
> *It's God knows when.*

> *From 60 to 70*
> *He still is inclined,*

But most of the time
It's a figment of mind.

From 70 to 80
He hopes it will last
And thinks it may be
A thing of the past

From 80 to 90
Although it's too late,
She still can remember
"That, honey, was great."

The truth is that penile rigidity and the force of ejaculation peak at approximately age seventeen. Men in their twenties and thirties require little sexual stimulation, and an erection will occur quickly and with very little prompting. Most men in this age group ejaculate relatively quickly. Another erection is possible within a brief period of time.

When men reach their forties they require more direct stimulation of the genitalia and perhaps some fantasy thoughts. An erection takes longer to develop and ejaculation and orgasm come more slowly. While another erection may occur, it usually takes significantly more time than when a man was in his twenties.

Men in their fifties and sixties require significantly greater amounts of direct stimulation of the genitalia. It takes longer to achieve an erection, and after ejaculation another erection may take a considerable period of time to develop.

Men in their seventies and eighties who are otherwise in good health can continue to have erections, although they may take longer to develop and may require more patience and great amounts of stimulation, and the erection may be less firm. Subsequent erections require a great deal more time to develop.

SEXUAL ADVANTAGES WITH AGING

The middle-aged and older male is stereotypically viewed as being sexually inadequate and unable to satisfy his female partner. Many younger men erroneously believe that their elders cannot participate in or enjoy sex. In truth, the middle-aged and older male may be better able to satisfy his female partner than his younger counterpart. Why is this so? Because by middle age the average man will be more sexually experienced and will usually know more sophisticated sexual techniques. He may be more attuned to satisfying his female partner and may engage in more imaginative foreplay. He may utilize different coital positions that are more stimulating and pleasing to the female. He may well be more emotionally involved in his sexual relationship.

Some of the physiological changes that occur with aging may in fact aid a male in satisfying his female partner. For example, the period of foreplay may last longer. This is important because it has been demonstrated that there is a relationship between the length of foreplay and the orgasmic response among females.

Another change that favors the older male is that the erection may be more prolonged before ejaculation occurs. Since there is a relationship between the duration of penetration and female orgasm, this again favors the older male.

Now that both men and women live longer than ever before, it is perhaps inevitable that preconceived notions exist concerning the sexual life of our senior citizens. Usually the older male is thought to have no sexual desire, and therefore it is assumed that if he is sexually active, he is a "dirty old man." Sometimes when an older man mentions his continuing sexual ability, people believe that he is engaging in wishful thinking.

The "golden years" of marriage have not been traditionally regarded as a time for sexual fulfillment. This period in a couple's relationship has been characterized by infrequent sexual activity. Many aging men believe that it is inevitable that they will become impotent. Many wives also expect a decrease in sexual ability on the part of their husbands as they age. Unfortunately, some physicians are misinformed about sex and aging and reinforce this belief. But loss of erection is not necessarily caused by the aging process. Older men do not necessarily lose interest in sex, and many continue to function actively. Our society should no longer view these men as abnormal but should encourage them, for it opens up another avenue of pleasure for older men and their partners. The sexually active older male is in fact generally a healthy individual.

It is of interest that males who experience sexual activity earlier in life and more frequently are more likely to retain their potency in later years.

It is noteworthy that when sexual relations between a couple do cease, women generally assign the responsibility for the cessation to their male partners. Interviews with men show that they also believe themselves to be the party most responsible for the discontinuation of sexual activity.

As medical progress continues to extend the life expectancy of our older citizens, and as new treatment modalities become available, sexual activity will become more common and accepted in older individuals. Men and their partners should not assume a defeatist attitude concerning sexual ability as they age, but should take heart in the adage that "the older the fiddle, the sweeter the tune."

18

IS THERE A MALE MENOPAUSE?

Only a fool never changes his mind.
—*Author unknown*

Key Points:

- Confusion exists as to whether there is a "menopause" in aging men.
- Testosterone levels do decrease with age.
- Libido may decrease with advancing years.
- Hormonal changes are generally not responsible for impotence.

One of the greatest fallacies concerning male impotence centers around the question of whether there is a male climacteric, or menopause. A few males will have symptoms similar to those experienced by menopausal females, such as nervousness, depression, lack of energy, and sometimes even hot flashes. However, this is not a common occurrence, and most impotence problems in this age group are not due to "male menopause."

In middle-aged women, there are very definite signs of physiological change. These include a decrease in the tone and size of the breasts and genitalia, a loss of feminine bodily contours, some deepening of the voice, and a tendency to grow more body hair. In the male, physiological changes are less apparent.

Testosterone, which is secreted primarily from the testicles and secondarily from the adrenal glands, is an important hormone in male development. It is known that testosterone levels are secreted in the male according to a circadian rhythm, with maximal levels occurring in the morning and minimal levels at night. It is also known that serum testosterone levels do decline with advancing age, beginning in the mid-forties. This is most likely a result of a decreased rate of production in the testicles due to aging. In addition, the size and weight of the testicles decrease with age. Seventy-year-old males may be expected to have approximately 50 percent of the testosterone concentrations found in men half their age.

However, almost all older men still have serum testosterone levels that are in a range considered to be normal, and testosterone levels in men who demonstrate varying levels of erectile ability usually fall within the normal range, indicating that testosterone itself is usually not a cause of impotence. But while low testosterone is generally not responsible for impotence, it may cause a loss of interest in sex.

As a man enters middle age, there are obvious changes in his emotional makeup. A man may realize for the first time that many of his early aspirations, either personal or occupational, will not be met. Other men feel that they have gone as far as they are going professionally and financially, and that there is really nothing to look forward to in life. These anxieties common to middle age may result in psychological impotence.

Many women state that they know their partner is going through a "change of life." But the fact is that this is probably not a physiological change but rather a psychological one.

Some men today believe they should be able to perform sexually like a machine. They expect that foreplay, erections, vaginal penetration, ejaculation, and orgasm will follow in an automatic sequence. Since most bodily functions, including sexual drive, vary from day to day, the chances of not living up to a predetermined standard are significant; therefore there is a great tendency for men, especially those of middle age, to believe that they are sexual underachievers. It is imperative that they and their female partners realize that sexual performance will vary from time to time and that there are no set standards that must be met on every occasion.

A sympathetic and considerate female partner is one of the most important factors in continuing potency in the male. Men and their partners should take heart in the knowledge that sex, like a fine wine, may improve with aging.

19

IS IT SAFE TO RESUME SEX AFTER A HEART ATTACK?

"The trouble is, Sancho," said Don Quixote, "you are
so afraid that you cannot see or hear properly: for
one of the effects of fear is to disturb the senses and
cause things to appear other than what they are."

—*Cervantes*

Key Points:

- Men who have had a heart attack may be afraid to resume sexual activity.
- The partners of heart attack patients may also be fearful of engaging in sex.
- Usually sexual intercourse is not an overly strenuous activity.
- Patients who have had heart attacks should seek guidance from their physicians.
- Most patients who have recovered from a heart attack can have an active sex life.

The male patient recovering from a heart attack is placed in a dependent position, since he now must rely heavily upon his family and friends, and certainly upon his physician. This dependence may diminish his feeling of masculinity. If his doctor does not bring up the matter of his future sexual life, he may conclude that intercourse is beyond his capability. Researchers have noted that two-thirds of patients who recover from a heart attack receive no sexual advice whatsoever from their physicians. In many of those cases in which advice is rendered, it is vague and not clearly understood.

A man convalescing from a heart attack often has a decreased libido. In addition, he may fear that he will die during intercourse in the "death in the saddle" manner. Many patients are hesitant to ask their physician's advice, either out of embarrassment or for fear of being told that their sexual life is over. Similarly, many wives are concerned with the situation but are reluctant to inquire because they do not want to put pressure on their husbands. Some women feel intercourse may cause too great a strain on their husband's heart and they withhold themselves, thereby increasing the male's frustration.

Studies reveal that few men resume normal sexual habits after a heart attack. Most have intercourse less frequently, and some abstain altogether. Does intercourse, in fact, impose a significant strain on the heart?

During intercourse the heart rate and oxygen consumption increase, and blood pressure rises. Physical demands peak at orgasm and decline slowly but steadily thereafter. Intercourse requires an average energy expenditure of approximately 150 calories. One can assess the physical work imposed by monitoring the heart rate, which is an indirect measurement of oxygen consumption. The pulse rate averages approximately 120 beats per minute at the time of orgasm. While this may seem to be a rather brisk rate, there is actually no more oxygen consumed than if one had quickly climbed two flights of steps. In short, physical exertion during intercourse is relatively low. Men expend approximately five calories per minute during sexual activity with a familiar partner. Compare that with four calories expended during a man's sleep. And one can reach five calories per minute expenditure by playing Ping-Pong, raking leaves, walking the course to play golf, or dancing. Sex has been calculated as being as strenuous as walking at a rate of 3.5 miles per hour.

Clearly, there are differences of opinion among physicians as to just how stressful sexual intercourse may be. The following anecdote humorously captures this difference.

A cardiologist, a resident training in cardiology, and an intern had a discussion concerning whether sexual intercourse was work or pleasure. The cardiologist said that in his opinion, sexual intercourse was approximately 60 percent work and 40 percent pleasure. The resident physician suggested that his experience was different; he considered intercourse to be approximately 40 percent work and 60 percent pleasure. Out of courtesy and in a condescending manner, they turned to the lowly intern, who had just spent most of the past year doing petty jobs for his mentors. He said, "You're both wrong! Intercourse is 100 percent pleasure, because if there were any work associated with it, I would be doing it for both of you."

The good news is that since sex is not an overly strenuous form of exercise, most men with heart disease can resume activity with a physician's guidance. Resumption of sexual activity may go hand in hand with a cardiac rehabilitation program. If a male is aware of any sexual techniques that seem to be too physically taxing, they should be avoided. For example, a male may be more comfortable lying on his back with his partner straddling him, since in this position the female performs most of the movement and the male does less thrusting. Exotic positions that require the male to support his partner's weight are probably best avoided.

Fear, usually resulting from lack of information, may cause men with coronary artery disease to avoid sex. This may manifest itself in a decrease either in sexual drive or in the ability to attain an erection. The good news is that armed with the above knowledge, many men will be able to resume sexual activity. It is advisable for both men and their partners to seek a physician's advice and guidance.

20

DEATH DURING INTERCOURSE

I am not afraid of death. I just don't want to be
there when it happens.

—*Woody Allen*

Key Points:

- Death during intercourse is a relatively uncommon event.
- Factors contributing are alcohol ingestion, food consumption,
  and an extramarital partner.

Should one worry about death during intercourse? In a Japanese
study of 5,559 cases of sudden death, thirty-four were noted to have
occurred during sexual intercourse, but only eighteen of these were
attributed to heart disease. Twenty-seven of the thirty-four deaths
occurred in association with an extramarital affair, which certainly
could be expected to impose more stress on the heart.

A pattern has been noted for men who died during intercourse. The
man is usually married and is with a woman not his wife, is in unfamil-
iar surroundings, and has recently consumed a large meal that included
alcohol.

While many believe that death during intercourse is the result of a
heart attack, this is not necessarily true. Heart attacks are generally
caused by blockage of blood flow in the arteries, usually from a buildup
of cholesterol. Death during intercourse is usually due to an arrhythmia,

which means that the normal rhythm of the beating heart is interrupted. Extreme irregularities in the heart rate and rhythm may cause it to cease function, thus resulting in death.

Physicians have evaluated patients with known coronary artery disease and checked their heart patterns while the patients wore ambulatory cardiac monitors. During intercourse the heart rate increased but was not significantly different from that noted during usual daily activities. While more than half of the men recorded extra beats, the same cardiac patterns were noted during other daily activities. And few of these cases included life-threatening arrhythmia. During intercourse there is also a rise in blood pressure and in the rate of respiration, both of which are generally well tolerated.

The truth is that heart attacks during sexual activity are a relatively rare event. Medical researchers reported on 858 sexually active men and women approximately a week after a heart attack. More than 80 percent of the patients studied were men. Only 0.9 percent reported having sexual activity within two hours of the onset of the heart attack. This translates into less than one heart attack in a hundred that can be related to sexual activity. The good news is that the risk for men with previously diagnosed coronary artery disease was just as low as for men who were apparently otherwise healthy. The researchers calculated that the risk of having a heart attack for a healthy fifty-year-old male in any given hour is one in a million. Sexual activity doubles the risk to two in a million. For men with known heart disease, the chances of having a heart attack while engaged in sexual activity is twenty in a million. With a properly supervised cardiac rehabilitation program, coupled with regular exercise, resumption of sexual activity by a patient with known heart disease is very reasonable. While sexual activity does increase the risk of a heart attack from approximately one in a million to two in a million, it is not a reason to avoid sex. Unfortunately, many men and their partners worry unjustifiably about this unlikely event. Before avoiding sex because of an unrealistic fear, patients and their partners should recall Mark Twain's statement: "My life has been filled with terrible things, most of which never happened to me."

While death during intercourse is really a rare event, some occurrences have made headlines. On January 26, 1979, at 10:15 p.m., in a townhouse at 13 West Fifty-fourth Street in New York City, Nelson Rockefeller, the man who had been governor of New York for fifteen years and vice president of the United States under Gerald Ford, and who was a grandson of the founder of Standard Oil, passed away. The only other person present at the time was a young woman named Megan Marshack. Marshack and Rockefeller allegedly were writing a book about his private art collection. Of interest is the fact that there were no papers present indicating their literary effort. However, on a table were food and wine. It is widely assumed that they were engaged in sexual intercourse.

Recognition that sexual intercourse is no more strenuous than climbing two flights of stairs, unless done outside of marital bonds, prompted the following verse written by a physician practicing internal medicine:

> *Coronary have a care,*
> *Think before that new affair.*
>
> *Domestic sex hardly makes you palpitate.*
> *Heartbeats stay at normal rate,*
> *When one beds with legal mate.*
>
> *And the dangers that it bears,*
> *Loom like—well, two sets of stairs.*
>
> *But roosting in another's nest,*
> *Flirts with cardiac arrest.*

Not to be outdone, another physician specializing in heart bypass surgery replied:

> *But if it's essential to indulge your lust,*
> *In the surgeon you can trust.*
>
> *To your oxygen-starved heart he'll bring*
> *The blood that's needed when you swing.*
>
> *You Don Juans need not despair*
> *Go ahead—have your affair.*
>
> *But keep in mind you risk your life,*
> *Because there is no surgical cure for the angry wife!*

21

IMPOTENCE AS A PREDICTOR OF HEART ATTACK AND STROKE

There was the Door to which I found no key;
There was the Veil through which I might not see.
—Omar Khayyám

Key Points:

- The onset of impotence may be a warning sign of cardiovascular disease.
- An impotent male should consider a cardiac evaluation.

The onset of impotence may be the first warning sign of a more serious underlying medical condition—a condition that could lead to a heart attack or stroke.

In 1990, in an article generally underappreciated by the medical community, the point was made that men who have no history of vascular disease of either the heart or brain but who have erection problems associated with poor blood flow to the penis are eight times more likely to suffer a attack and five times more likely to experience a stroke within 24 to 36 months of the onset of impotence than males who have no such problem. Thus, erectile insufficiency may be a signal for men to have a vascular evaluation to assess blood flow to the heart and brain. The ability to attain and sustain an erection may be a barometer of a man's general vascular health. If one views the penis as an organ in itself, just like the heart and brain, it is easier to understand that poor blood flow to the penis may indicate poor or reduced blood flow to the heart and brain.

Studies of men recovering from heart attacks in coronary care units reveal that more than half the patients report impotence as a problem *prior* to their heart attack.

The good news is that certain risk factors that may impact negatively on blood flow to the heart and brain, as well as the penis, can be modified. These factors include high blood pressure (hypertension), cigarette smoking, obesity, a fatty diet, and insufficient exercise.

Keeping one's blood pressure stabilized, avoiding cigarettes, exercising regularly, and eating a low-fat diet may all contribute to maintaining erectile ability. A man's desire to maintain sexual potency may be a greater motivator to follow a healthy lifestyle than fear of a future heart attack or stroke.

22

DOES BIKE RIDING CAUSE IMPOTENCE?

Every man is entitled to his own opinion. No man is
entitled to base his opinion upon the wrong facts.

—*Bernard Baruch*

Key Points:

- Pressure on the artery to the penis from a bike seat may reduce blood flow.
- Straddle injuries from the bike's tubular bar may cause impotence.
- It has been suggested, but not yet proved, that bike riding may cause impotence in males.
- It has been hypothesized that bike riding may cause excessive pressure on the female anatomy and cause problems with clitoral response.

This question has caused a ripple of concern within the bicycle riding community. Dr. Irwin Goldstein, a prominent urologist in Boston and one of the world's leaders in research on impotence, suggests that riding bicycles may, in fact, cause impotence. And there is supporting data. A study in Boston shows that impotence is more common in bikers than runners. In a survey of running and cycling clubs, 1.1 percent of runners reported impotence as compared to 4.2 percent of bikers. Both groups were in good physical condition.

The blood vessels that supply the penis are located in the perineum (the area between the base of the scrotum and the rectum). A bicycle seat may apply excess pressure to these important blood vessels. If pressure from a bike seat does, in fact, reduce blood flow to the penis and if this in turn causes impotence, there is still an important question. How much riding is necessary before a problem develops? Since the reduced flow and the impotence, if it in fact occurs, may come on gradually, it is very difficult to know.

Most men are aware of certain discomforts, such as "saddle soreness," that come from bike riding. However, if a male begins to experience numbness in the penis or scrotum, this may be a warning sign of excessive pressure. Most bike riders are aware that if they dismount, a normal feeling and sensation will return within a matter of minutes.

There are several ways to lessen the chance of developing a problem with potency. These include dismounting on a regular basis to relieve pressure on the artery; not extending the legs, since extension places more weight on the bike seat; and directing the nose of the seat downward a few degrees. Because heavier men may be at greater risk of compression of blood flow, they should take extra caution. The pressure can be relieved by using a wider bicycle seat. Fortunately, the bicycle industry is responding, and now there are several types of seats that are designed to lessen the risk of injury to the blood supply to the penis.

There is another form of injury that is of more acute onset. This is a straddle injury, caused by striking the top tube. When selecting a bike, one should be certain that the tube is designed low enough so that when the rider mounts the bike, the tube is several inches below the perineum.

In all cases, cyclists should avoid large bumps, which may cause increased pressure. This is particularly true since mountain biking has become so popular. Shock absorbers on the seat or the rear part of the chassis may reduce impact.

Dr. Goldstein has also raised an intriguing question about whether bicycling can cause a problem with sexual function in women. He notes that the nerve and blood supply to the clitoris also run in the perineum, and he has early data suggesting that some bike riders complain of a problem with clitoral function.

Another question yet to be answered is that if pressure from bicycle seats causes penile and clitoral problems, is it reversible if one gives up bike riding? Clearly, more research is needed. Dr. Goldstein has stated, "I cannot say that sitting on a bicycle seat causes impotence but I can go on record with supporting data to show that sitting on a bicycle seat compresses the artery." However, following the advice above may prevent any potential problem.

23

THE SINGLE MAN AND SEX

Men say: "Let's make love and things will be better."
Women say: "Let's make things better, then we'll
make love."

—*Julian Slowinski, Psy.D.*

Key Points:

- Single men have to face a special set of circumstances to remain sexually healthy.
- Impotence can be either primary (never having a successful attempt at intercourse) or secondary (occurring after a history of successful intercourse), and it can be related to a number of causes.
- Men need to know what turns them on sexually in order to give their erectile capacity the best chance to function. This is especially important for single men with erectile difficulties.
- When a single man is getting to know a potential sexual partner, his worst enemy is worrying about his future sexual performance.
- Sexual success can benefit from a little bit of luck.

Sex for the single man presents a special set of potential difficulties, whether that man is straight, gay, or bisexual. For the single man, establishing and maintaining a sexual relationship may involve some anxiety and trials of confidence. This can be true whether he is unattached and just looking for a partner or has just separated from a relationship through breakup, divorce, or death. The issues of sexual performance and functioning are the same. Can he deal with the potential anxiety of sex with a new partner and have his erections behave as they should?

In earlier chapters, we have referred to many issues that contribute to erectile failure. All of the psychological and interpersonal issues we mentioned apply to single men as well as men already in relationships or marriages. Performance anxiety, spectatoring, conflicts about being sexual, sexual scripting, and sexual self-image can all influence the sexual functioning of the single man. But unlike men with regular partners, the unattached male is in many ways more vulnerable to the self-defeating cycle of repeated erectile failure with each new partner. He can often suffer a decrease in sexual confidence without the benefit of a committed and understanding partner. Given his own personality issues and degree of sexual disappointment, he may withdraw from sexual activity altogether, or seek gratification in masturbation and other solitary pursuits.

As we have stated before, for the sake of diagnostic clarification, therapists and physicians describe both *primary* impotence (men who have never been able to maintain an erection sufficient for penetration during an attempt at intercourse) and *secondary* impotence (men who develop erectile problems after a history of successful completions of intercourse). These diagnostic labels are not meant to imply that one is more serious than the other. The causes, consequences, and treatments can be similar. The history and examination of the man's erectile problem usually will clarify whether the causes are physical, psychological, or a combination.

Tony is a twenty-five-year-old bachelor who is likable and outgoing and has a good job in the computer industry. He still lives at home with his parents, saying that he can save money and he enjoys his mother's cooking. Despite his active interest in dating, Tony has never been successful in attempts at intercourse with women. Tony is easily aroused, and his erections are fine, but he loses his erection each time he attempts penetration. Some of the women he has dated have been understanding and supportive, but Tony's embarrassment and growing sense of helplessness have resulted in his avoiding sex and dating for some time. He now seeks sexual outlet through masturbation and getting aroused at striptease bars. Tony feels trapped in his current lifestyle and has almost written off trying to resume a sexual relationship with a partner.

There may be a simple explanation. The man like Tony who is dealing with primary erectile difficulties may just be dealing with performance anxiety and may merely need to be reassured that all can be well for him. Recall our discussion of the PLISSIT model of intervening in sexual complaints. Sometimes the simplest explanation and intervention is the best and most helpful. There are other times when the reason for erectile failure is more complicated. The man's response to erectile failures may bring up other issues that need attention and exploration.

As a partial list, many sexual difficulties including erectile problems, could be related to any or some of the following items:

1. Negative attitudes about sex and being sexual
2. Negative or ambivalent attitudes about women
3. Religious guilt about sex
4. Confusion about sexual orientation
5. Negative attitudes about homosexual sex (if gay)
6. Fear of intimacy and potential commitment to a partner
7. Negative family scripts about sex and emotional involvement
8. Poorly developed or inadequate interpersonal or social dating skills
9. Ignorance about basic sexual skills
10. Inadequate or inappropriate patterns of arousal without a partner
11. Issues related to earlier sexual abuse

It is worth repeating that issues on this list can play a part in both primary and secondary erectile difficulties. Most of the items listed are self-explanatory, while others need to be spelled out in more detail. There can also be an interplay between possible causes. For example, religious guilt and negative family scripts can foster the negative attitude that sex for pleasure is something "sinful." For some men, "waiting until marriage" solves the problem, and sexual functioning is fine when the union occurs in conjunction with social acceptance. For others, the anxiety about sex is so deep that even the blessing of the church or synagogue and family do not provide enough permission to be free to be sexually responsive.

For some men, erectile failure stirs up issues of sexual orientation. There are several potential explanations behind this concern. A man with difficulties may believe the sexual myth that "if you have trouble functioning with a woman, you must be gay," and worry that "you never know about these things." Or there may in fact be issues about sexual orientation that failed attempts at heterosexual intercourse bring to the surface. Or a man may truly be gay, but be so homophobic that he cannot deal with honestly exploring his sexual orientation.

Gay men with erectile difficulties need adequate therapeutic attention. For the single gay man there is a particular emphasis placed on having good erections. An inability to function not only brings the expected psychological stresses of dealing with impotence, but potentially places him in a passive role in sexual encounters. Being a passive recipient may prevent him from feeling like an equal partner. This can lead to self-esteem issues if he is uncomfortable with a passive role. In committed relationships, however, this may not be as much a problem, as pleasing the partner may be a real and enjoyed priority. In addition, if he is not practicing safe sex, a gay single male who is repeatedly a passive partner may also be placing himself at greater risk for contracting a sexually transmitted disease.

Being sexual with a partner requires a number of responses and skills, including both feeling desire for that partner, being aroused by that partner, and being able to kindle sexual response in that partner. There are some men who develop a regular pattern of sexual arousal through masturbation or fantasy that they cannot transfer to a sexual partner. If they are not aroused with a partner, they can fail to obtain or maintain an erection. For example, their masturbation practice might not involve even touching their penis. For them masturbation may consist of lying on their stomach and rubbing their penis (erect or not erect) against the bed or some object. Having orgasms on a regular basis with a flaccid penis does not train a man for good erections with a partner. In addition, such men may find that being touched by a partner may not be sufficiently arousing to provide an erection.

Some men may use adult films as a vehicle for sexual arousal. While this practice may help in enhancing their sex lives, the use of explicit sexual materials or pornography as the sole outlet for sexual enjoyment can result in men distancing themselves from interaction with true sexual partners. An exclusive use of these materials can interfere with a single man's openness to the behavioral and emotional interplay that occurs between sexual partners. As a consequence, when some of these men are faced with a "real-life" partner, they may have difficulty becoming sufficiently aroused for sex. They are not used to the cues and responses that are fostered by a relationship. The situation is a bit like the old saying "You have to be able to receive love in order to give love," or "You have to be able to give to get." Being able to be tuned in to a partner is very important for a successful sexual encounter and relationship.

Some men have conditioned themselves to become aroused to certain fantasies or use of fetish objects, so that sex with a partner without meeting certain erotic conditions (such as her wearing "sexy underwear," or him being "cross-dressed") may not result in arousal sufficient for him to obtain or maintain an erection.

Another example of the use of a solitary form of arousal is the practice of anonymous phone sex or computer chat lines. Again, these vehicles for sexual gratification allow arousal to be achieved without the potential embarrassment of dealing face to face with a partner. For some men, the habit of seeking these readily available avenues of solitary sexual gratification can lead to performance difficulties when they are actually with a partner. Others will successfully use these experiences to fuel arousal fantasies when they are with a partner. Men who confine their sexual practices exclusively to the use of these solitary means of gratification are really avoiding the potential performance anxiety of being sexual with a partner. (However, certain sex therapy techniques for the treatment of erectile disorders do encourage the active use of fantasy in order to reduce anxiety and build confidence. This is an accepted clinical practice and is not at all related to the exclusive type of solitary practice that we are discussing.)

Any of these situations just mentioned can underlie both primary and secondary erectile difficulties and will require therapeutic attention. These men may need to learn to develop arousal patterns involving more "appropriate" objects of their erotic attention in order to function better with a partner. There are times when a partner is glad or at least willing to participate in a particular sexual practice in order to allow the male to be aroused to complete intercourse. Sometimes this level of cooperation works. At other times the participation is at the increasing expense of the partner's enjoyment of sex. We said earlier that sex is never simple.

TREATMENT FOR SINGLES

The single man who is experiencing secondary erectile difficulties with a new partner may be affected by issues of loyalty to a former partner, or even anger and distrust of a previous lover that make being open to a new person more difficult. Anxiety about potential emotional intimacy in a new relationship can be directly transferred to an inhibition of genital response. The contributing causes are usually easily accessible with some exploration. What remains is an awareness of the ingredients that the individual man needs in order to feel comfortable in the new relationship. This includes having a supportive partner and being free from anxiety about adequate functioning. Sometimes, treatment for these single men can be brief, supportive, and to the point. It involves eliminating negative thinking, reducing performance anxiety, and enhancing patterns of arousal with new partners. Successful treatment also builds on past success to restore confidence. At other times, the episode of transitory impotence requires therapy to explore sex-related issues that may have existed for a lifetime and could have been an issue in previous relationships.

The single man who has never been able to function adequately with a sexual partner will require both similar and additional therapeutic attention. Individual therapy may be indicated to explore causes of the difficulty. Relaxation training and the practice of imagery of successful sexual functioning will be helpful, as will masturbation training to rehearse and encourage appropriate patterns of arousal. The acquisition of better interpersonal social skills, including assertiveness training, may be indicated, in addition to correcting areas of sexual ignorance through education.

The unavailability of a regular sexual partner can also contribute to erectile problems for a single male. It is not easy to meet someone new, establish a relationship, and move toward a sexual experience while at the same time worrying about sexual failure. The use of sexual surrogates in sex therapy is not always an available option. A single male is fortunate if he has a person or friend available who would be willing to help as a "temporary partner" in overcoming his erectile difficulties. Even if this is a possibility, there is still the question of whether sexual success gained this way will provide a man with enough confidence to transfer his experience to a new partner.

Whenever a man who has been experiencing erectile difficulties meets a potential partner, it is important for him to proceed slowly and develop a trusting and supportive relationship. On the other hand, there will always be some men who meet the right partner, under the right circumstances, and immediately move to an instant cure—successful sex! A little luck can't hurt.

Finally, but not at all last, is the use of medical intervention to assist the single male. The most recent developments in overcoming impotence, including Viagra, injections, transurethral pellets, the vacuum pump, and surgical implants, do not require the direct cooperation of a sexual partner. The confidence that is inspired in a male who knows that his erection can be assisted through pharmacological or mechanical intervention may be all that he needs to resume the level of functioning that is normal for him. Unfortunately, many men mistakenly feel that all it will take is the correct prescription to make erectile difficulties a thing of the past. The reality is that not all men are helped by all of the new treatments for impotence. For example, preexisting medical conditions and/or the current use of certain medications may make the use of the current impotence drugs ineffective or unsafe. The advice of a physician is needed to determine who will benefit from the proper use of these new medications for erectile difficulties.

24

SEXUALITY AND RELIGION

Oh that you would kiss me with the kisses of your
mouth! For your love is better than wine.
—*Song of Solomon, 1:1–2*

Key Points:

- Even nonreligious people are affected by religious attitudes about sexuality.
- Many people take it for granted that organized religions are sex-negative in attitude and teachings.
- Many religious denominations are evolving toward an understanding of the nature of human sexuality.
- Many men are anxious about experiencing sexual pleasure because of their early understanding of religious attitudes about sexual expression.

RELIGIOUS INFLUENCES ON SEXUAL ATTITUDES AND FUNCTIONING: IS THERE A PROBLEM?

Religion is a fact of life, even if we choose to ignore it. We all have a religious history, whether it be observant, nonpracticing, indifferent, or oppositional. Most religious systems speak to the same human issues of intimacy and sexuality from their own view and traditions. Religious values in our culture still have enormous impact on the attitudes and psychological responses to sexual feelings and behaviors, even among "nonreligious" people. And at times the messages we receive from our religious traditions are confusing and contradictory.

What is a person to do? Unfortunately, many people feel that their sexual life and their early religious beliefs about sexuality are incompatible. They struggle to reconcile their earlier religious training and experiences with their current understanding of their own sexuality. They recognize the prominent influence of their early training on their thinking and behavior patterns, and how it affects their overall sexual relationships. These same men and women often see little sense in turning to their "sex-negative" denominations for clarity on teachings about sex. In a sense, many adults are trying to live their sexual lives armed with a grammar-school understanding of their particular faith's teaching and attitudes about sexuality. They share with the general public a superficial knowledge about religion and sexuality and bear the impact of erroneous beliefs on their minds and behavior. They are also confused about what to tell the next generation about the interface between human sexuality and religious belief. And so it continues, from generation to generation. Yes, there is a problem with religion and sexuality. It does not have to remain that way.

THE BIBLE AND BEYOND

We can better understand the dilemma that many people face about religion and sex if we take a moment to consider the tradition we have inherited. Many people look to the Bible for guidance about what constitutes proper behavior. While it is true that some religious denominations draw their traditional teachings about sexuality directly, and even exclusively, from scripture, there is not total agreement on this among denominations. For example, there are faith groups that rely on the Bible as a foundation, but also have developed a tradition that includes teachings that reflect an evolving and informed understanding of human sexuality. As a result, different denominations, and their respective clergy and members, may come to hold various opinions and understandings of the meaning and application of scriptural passages and teachings. Many scripture scholars would argue that the Bible is not a code book for sexual ethics, and would advise us not to look for answers in Biblical texts that may not be there. Such a view can lead, for example, to a variety of understandings about issues such as male and female gender roles, masturbation, homosexuality, birth control, abortion, the use of erotica, and premarital and extramarital sex. The reality is that within and between religious groups there is more than just one way to understand the nature, purpose, and function of human sexuality.

Many men and women are confused about or are not aware of various schools of thought about sexual matters even within their own denomination. They are more or less accepting of common interpretations, and may feel they have no choice other than uncritical acceptance or outright rejection of their religious belief about sex. Some end up "throwing out the baby with the bathwater." As we have stated, many people are trying to live adult sexual lives armed with only a grammar-school understanding of sex and religion. In many cases, people internalize and assume a rather "sex-negative" outlook that is often based on a misunderstanding of religious teachings. People have learned to distrust sexual feelings and associate guilt with pleasure. As we will see shortly, this can often lead to difficulties in sexual functioning.

It becomes easy to see that what we have received in our diverse society is a long-standing tradition that tends to resist biologically natural responses in the name of religious and cultural teachings. It is not surprising that many men and women have difficulty making a transition to enjoying a sexual union that has been blessed by their religious denomination and their society. After years of negative and double messages about the underside of sex, some people cannot make the switch to being carefree and guiltless. They may feel that their denomination has sacramentally or ritualistically sanitized sex via marriage, but the early messages linger and can affect healthy functioning. Some men and women still distrust their normal sexual feelings as being at least suspect or partially sinful. Do not enjoy sex too much! Dualism, the split between the body and the spirit, lives! Even in more liberal denominations, sexual expression can remain somewhat suspect, and matters of the spirit are elevated as being better or more pure. Religious role models still exist that emphasize chastity and abstinence (for reasons other than the avoidance of disease and pregnancy), and by implication suggest that we would be better off if we transcended our sexual nature. Rather than have the erotic nature of men and women take a backseat to matters of the spirit, one would hope instead for balance and inclusiveness.

WHAT THERAPISTS OFTEN SEE

Therapists are well aware that anxiety and fear generated from early attitudes and sexual experiences can contribute to adult sexual dysfunction. Men and women still report to therapists their sense of guilt and discomfort about sexual feelings, sexual desire, and sexual pleasure that are not caused by other emotional problems. At times, the discomfort that is reported is related to common sexual practices that their religion viewed with disapproval. For example, masturbation, oral sex, birth control, homosexuality, and abortion, while not equivalent practices, often cause considerable conflict. Some people attribute religious guilt to sexual activities merely because they are pleasurable! As one otherwise well-educated woman told her therapist: "But they told us that our vaginas would burn in hell for all eternity if we touched ourselves."

THE PROBLEM OF DESIRE: A CLINICAL EXAMPLE

Guilt and anxiety about sexual feelings and behavior can affect both men and women at any stage of the sexual response cycle. We also know that difficulties in one area can lead to problems in another. For example, inhibited sexual desire can lead to both inhibited arousal and erectile dysfunction. As an example, let us focus on sexual desire difficulties in men (and women too) that can be attributed to a sex-negative religious experience and that are commonly seen by sex therapists. As we pointed out earlier in the book, a primary task of psychological development is becoming aware of one's sexual feelings and understanding them as natural and as a part of the sense of self. While sexual feeling are biologically programmed, it is the socialization and control of them by religious and cultural norms that fill the experience, acceptance, and expression of sexual feeling with special meaning. It is the meaning, or personal psychological value, given to sexual desire that can prompt confusion in people.

If we feel that desire equals sin, then sexual desire can become a natural experience that can lead to anticipatory anxiety rather than to pleasure. In order to avoid this discomfort, a man might suppress his sexual feeling to the point where he also inhibits his desire for sex. In other words, a man (or woman) can become uncomfortable with internal feelings of sexual desire, label those natural desires as morally wrong, and feel guilty for what is really a genetically programmed response. As a result, the man may suppress sexual expression or deny the normal pleasure associated with sexual feelings. Erectile failure is a common response, if he should attempt to engage in sexual activity.

For many people, sexual desire and arousal can lead to anxiety and guilt. (The term "guilty masturbator" applies here.) Distrust of his own sexual pleasure can also prevent a man from responding to his sexual partner. This pattern is also frequently seen in women who shut down their orgasmic response as a reaction to a guilt-induced anxiety generated by mounting sexual arousal. Are these men (and women) punishing themselves for desiring forbidden fruit? We cannot prove it. We do know that erections are very sensitive to religious guilt. It is the same guilt over enjoying sexual pleasure that is the reason why some men (and women) are not satisfied with their sexual lives, even if they function without difficulty. The root of difficulties that lie in religious prohibitions needs to be addressed as part of treatment and should not be taken lightly. Not everyone who suffers from religion-induced sexual guilt can take the simple advice that one "shouldn't pay attention to such old fashioned notions." For many people, religion and sex are a very complicated issue. Sex is never simple.

THERAPY AS A POSITIVE INFLUENCE

Dealing with religiously based sexual difficulties can present a problem for therapists as well as the patient. Not all therapists are exposed to dealing with religious issues as part of their general training. Many feel that dealing with these questions is more the role of the clergy, and perhaps this is true, particularly in clarifying the teachings of a particular denomination. However, we know that many people are reluctant to discuss sexual matters with a member of the clergy, either out of embarrassment or out of fear of getting a standard "party line" response that may not address their needs on the matter. If a referral to a member of the clergy is made by a therapist, it should be to a cleric who is also aware of, and even sympathetic to, current psychosexual issues. He or she can then provide a more informed consultation. It is often helpful for the therapist and member of the clergy to work collaboratively in guiding the patient through the questions and issues that are interfering with sexual health.

As for the specific role of the therapist, he or she can be of great assistance in clarifying, understanding, questioning, and exploring the nature of the issues resolved in the religious conflict that can underlie so many sexual difficulties. Sexual guilt can often be assuaged by imparting accurate clinical information about, for example, the "normalcy" of sexual desire, the common occurrence of masturbation and oral sex, and the role of sexual fantasy as natural human function. Therapy can teach men (and women) to explore the basis of their religious/sexual beliefs and to respectfully challenge their often uninformed and even irrational notions that are interfering with their sexual functioning. These important concepts need to be explored, for the treatment of erectile failure and other sexual dysfunctions often include the use of sexual fantasy, erotic materials, and masturbation exercises. One does not want to have treatment cause more problems for the person because of an inappropriate intervention.

The process of dealing with questions of sex and religion can take time and will often include assignments for outside reading. These may include readings in basic sexuality education, or even specific referral to contemporary Biblical scholarship. These resources are particularly helpful when dealing with matters of sexual orientation, whether it is of primary concern to the patient or is directly related to a specific sexual dysfunction. Of course, treatment recommendations are made only after careful exploration with the patient. The therapist should always be mindful to respect and be guided by the firmly held beliefs of those seeking treatment. Everyone proceeds at his—or her—own pace.

IS THERE HOPE FOR RELIGION AND SEX?

Yes, there are new trends toward healthier religious understanding of the role of human sexuality. Religious teaching need not lead to guilt and sexual problems. Just as there are many nonreligious people who have sexual difficulties, so there are many religiously observant men and women who do not have sexual problems. Many contemporary religious writers are taking a new look at traditional attitudes, aided by modern advances in social science and contemporary studies in scripture and ethics. Rather than focusing on moral absolutes, theologians and ethicists are paying increased attention to a holistic understanding of sexuality. This focus places value on intimate relationships characterized by mutual respect, freedom, personal growth, and integration. A holistic approach to understanding the person's sexual nature is not as centered on "acts" (e.g., it's a sin to touch yourself; or certain thoughts are "dirty" and therefore "sinful"), but rather on personal acceptance and responsible relationships. This approach makes sense to many who would be otherwise mired in guilt or feel alienated because of a personal inability to follow or accept traditional teachings (as is often the case for those coping with issues such as contraception, abortion, and homosexual orientation.) The new religious thinking is an attempt to move away from a destructive sexual ethic that far too often resulted in frustration and alienation. This is not to imply that a holistic vision of human sexuality means that "anything goes." There are still expectations about the limits of personal freedom and the need for responsible behavior. No one has yet to throw out the Ten Commandments!

Many men (and women) mired down by their grammar-school understanding of their sexual and religious past might find that an exploration of more contemporary religious approaches to sexuality helps to clarify the issue and allow them to be sexual and discover the real pleasure of guilt-free sexual intimacy. For others, merely having a better awareness of the early origins of religious understanding of sexuality enables them to conclude for themselves what weight to place on these beliefs in their own life.

What is important to gain from this brief overview is the powerful impact of religious beliefs and values on our culture and attitudes about sexuality. These values are deeply ingrained and can influence us, whether we are committed believers, casually observant, or nonbelievers. The important fact remains that religion can be a positive influence for those people who respect and need the structure and the comfort of feeling within a supportive ethical system.

Many religious systems are becoming much more "sex-positive" in their approach to understanding human sexuality. Many people would be pleasantly surprised (or shocked) to find that their own denomination has come a long way in expanding its view of human sexuality since their childhood. There may no longer be the need to live one's adult sexual life guided by a grammar-school understanding of one's religious attitude toward sex. Things may have changed. In truth, many people were not paying attention. For others, the sex-positive evolution of religious understanding will be a needed support.

For some people, religion will always be an issue of concern and confusion in their sexual lives. Others will be motivated to expand their religious understanding to incorporate new and refreshing ideas. And there are those for whom the whole topic is not a consideration at all. Everyone is different and will seek his—or her—own level of comfort.

25

HOW OFTEN DOES THE AVERAGE MAN HAVE INTERCOURSE?

Gentleman, there are three kinds of lies—lies, damned lies, and statistics.

—Disraeli

Key Points:

A recent survey reveals that adults average fifty-eight sexual episodes per year.

- Above-average sexual activity was noted in individuals who are:

  Married,
  Have children,
  Work long hours.

- Above-average sexual activity was also seen in:

  Jazz fans,
  Gun owners,
  Those with liberal political views.

- One in five adults has not engaged in any sexual activity during the previous year.
- Fifteen percent of adults engage in half of all sexual activity.
- Forty-two percent of adults account for 85 percent of all sex.

continued on next page

Key Points (cont.):

- Sexual activity decreases with age. Above age seventy-five, 8 percent of men and women account for 85 percent of all sexual activity.
- Men and women with the most education have the least sexual activity.
- Catholics are more sexually active than Protestants. Jews and agnostics are more sexually active than either Christian group.
- More sexually active individuals than sexually inactive individuals tend to report a happier marriage and happier life in general.
- None of the data presented should be used to compare yourself for purposes of determining if you are "normal."

A question not infrequently asked by men being evaluated at sexual dysfunction clinics is what the "normal" frequency of intercourse is. Many men who are having sexual difficulties focus on how often, or infrequently, they engage in intercourse. Some men's misconceptions impose further unnecessary pressures upon an already frustrating situation.

It is with considerable reservation and reluctance that data are offered below. The numbers may send the wrong message to males who are already overly concerned about their sexual inadequacy. The truth is that the frequency of intercourse is strictly couple-dependent. What is too often for one couple may be too infrequent for another. If a woman desires sexual intercourse nearly every day and her male partner is satisfied with having sex only twice a week, he may seem inadequate to her. On the other hand, another woman with a much lower sexual appetite might find intercourse twice a week to be too much. When a couple's desires are widely divergent, the relationship is threatened. In his classic work *Psychopathia Sexualis*, Richard Krafft-Ebing describes one man who "appeared, according to the statement of his wife, in the whole time of their married life covering a period of twenty-eight years, hypersexual, extremely libidinous, ever potent, in fact insatiable in his marital relations. During coitus he became quite bestial and wild, trembled all over with excitement and panted heavily. This nauseated the wife, who, by nature, was rather frigid, and rendered the discharge of her conjugal duty a heavy burden."

Another reason one hesitates to give statistical data is that no one is really certain how many times a week the average male has intercourse. Statistics are difficult to collect, since many people are reluctant to provide this information, and much of what has been obtained may be exaggerated. However, the data below are offered for several reasons. It exists, and it is of interest to many men, although of much less concern to most women. We hope that men will not focus on numbers, will regard this information as being simply of general interest, and will remember that numbers based on surveys have no meaning to an individual couple.

The frequency of sexual intercourse varies with age. As we would expect, younger groups tend to be more sexually active than older groups. For example, one study, by Carl Pearlman, showed that up to age thirty, approximately 44 percent of all men have intercourse three to four times a week, and at least 30 percent have intercourse one to two times a week. Between the ages of fifty and sixty, only 5 percent have intercourse three to four times a week, and 16 percent have it one to two times a week. In the eighth decade, less than 1 percent have intercourse three to four times a week, and less than 5 percent one to two times a week.

Many people believe that single men are more sexually active than married men, and that they engage in sexual activity whenever possible. However, studies indicate that married men are more active sexually. Between the ages of twenty and twenty-nine, 45 percent of married men have intercourse three to four times a week, while only 12 percent of single men have intercourse this often. Interestingly, divorced men are more sexually active at those same ages than either single or married men.

In a very revealing survey published by *Playboy* magazine in October 1973, more than two thousand people in twenty-four cities and suburban areas were interviewed. The article showed that since Dr. Alfred Kinsey's epic report on male sexual behavior more than twenty-five years before, there had been a general increase in the frequency of sexual intercourse. In Kinsey's studies, the median frequency of sexual intercourse for married couples twenty-five years of age or younger was about 130 times a year, while more recent estimates had risen to approximately 154 times per year. For ages thirty-six to forty-five, the median frequency of sexual intercourse noted by Kinsey was seventy-five times a year, while more recently it had risen to ninety-nine. For married people beyond their mid-fifties, the median had increased from twenty-six to forty-nine times per year.

It is generally recognized that one's early sexual activity normally affects one's later sexual behavior. Generally speaking, men who engage in sexual intercourse at an early age tend to participate in sexual intercourse longer than those men who began their sexual activity later.

More recent data come from scientists at the University of Chicago. General findings are that American adults have intercourse on an average approximately fifty-eight times a year. Groups reporting above-average sexual activity include those who are married, have little free time, have children at home, and work longer than average hours.

Other men who experience above-average sexual activity include those who have liberal political views, are owners of guns, or are jazz fans. Men who are more educated, especially those who have attended graduate school, are less sexually active than men with less education. This is true for women too. Why increasing education is associated with a decline in sexual frequency is unclear. Demographers also noted a correlation between the level of sexual activity and religious preference. Catholics are more active in general than Protestants but have sex less frequently than either Jews or agnostics. Baptists are more active than either Presbyterians or Lutherans.

Perhaps not so surprising is the finding that the most sexually active males are more likely to approve of premarital and extramarital sex and express a greater interest in pornography.

Other important findings are that people who are more sexually active report having a happier life and marriage than those who engage less often in sex. Those who feel life is interesting and exciting have more intercourse than those who feel life is generally boring. This raises the question of whether increased sexual activity makes one happier or whether happy people tend to engage more frequently.

Perhaps not surprising is the fact that the frequency of sexual intercourse is not evenly distributed among men. Fifteen percent of males account for about half of all sexual activity and approximately 40 percent of men are responsible for 85 percent of sexual activity. Keep in mind that sex is not the only thing that is spread unevenly in our population. Twenty percent of Americans possess half of all the money and 15 percent of the population consumes 85 percent of the wine.

We often try to determine who has the highest rate of intercourse. But what about numbers pertaining to sexual inactivity? About 20 percent of both men and women acknowledge that they had no sexual activity in the prior year.

As expected, the University of Chicago survey noted that the frequency of sexual activity is greatest in men in their twenties and thirties and gradually declines thereafter. The most rapid decrease is seen in men who are sixty-five and older.

It is important to maintain perspective. Surveys, no matter how well controlled, represent but a sampling of a given population on a particular subject. Despite the validity conferred by statistical tests, all combinations and permutations of behavior cannot be assessed or measured. The behavior of a few members of any species does not necessarily represent the behavior of all members, any more than one lion can represent a pride, one goose a gaggle, one fish a school, one whale a pod, or one ferret a business.

The above data should be regarded as points of interest rather than as guidelines for the normal frequency of intercourse. It is neither possible nor important to come up with exact numbers. It is much more important that both partners in a relationship be satisfied.

26

CAN THE PENIS BE LENGTHENED? DOES IT SHRINK? WILL IT BREAK?

If a man could have half his wishes, he would double his troubles.

—*Author unknown*

Key Points:

- The penis cannot be lengthened significantly.
- The penis does not shrink significantly.
- The penis can fracture.

Certain questions arise often enough that they deserve discussion. They are asked by both impotent men and those who are having no problem with sexual functioning. Some are interested for personal reasons; others are just curious. Most are misinformed. The true answers follow.

CAN THE PENIS BE LENGTHENED?

Some members of the medical profession, generally regarded as unscrupulous by their colleagues, have advertised that they can increase the length of the penis. Despite various surgical procedures, most patients do not gain any significant length, and a one-inch gain is considered a dramatic success. Increase in girth of the penis, between one to two inches, is achievable by transferring fat from another part of the body to the penis. However, much of the fat is later reabsorbed and repeat treatments will be necessary. In addition, the penis may assume a deformed shape.

The quality of the result is clearly subjective. One urologist rendering a second opinion on the surgical outcome achieved by one of his colleagues described the penis as looking like a misshapen kielbasa.

Some patients who have undergone surgery become "penis cripples" and suffer psychologically from the deformity that can follow. This type of surgery has led to many malpractice actions against urologists, and some have lost their license to practice medicine. Such procedures should be avoided!

While modern medicine has made great strides in transplanting various organs, including the heart, lungs, kidney, pancreas, and portions of the eye, a penis transplant today is not a practical matter. Not only would one be confronted with the problem of rejection of the tissue because it is foreign to the recipient, but it is very difficult to imagine who would volunteer to be the donor.

Claims have been made that vacuum pumps designed to help achieve an erection, which are discussed in detail in Chapter 13, may also be effective in achieving penile enlargement. The pumps do help impotent males achieve an erection, but there are no data to indicate that the length or girth of the penis is increased significantly by their use.

As discussed in Chapter 7, "Myths and Fallacies," penile length is not usually an issue for female satisfaction.

DOES THE PENIS SHRINK?

The penis may become temporarily smaller after exposure to cold. This change is transient and disappears under normal temperature conditions. With aging or following castration, which may have been done to treat prostate cancer, there may be some decrease in size. However, in many cases this is more apparent than real. Most middle-aged and older men who complain that their penis is getting smaller have really simply gained weight and the more protuberant lower abdomen gives the appearance of a shorter penis.

An interesting phenomenon exists concerning males who believe the penis is shrinking—the "Koro syndrome." Koro is an unusual and extreme form of anxiety that leaves the male with the firm belief that his penis is suddenly shrinking and will disappear. This condition occurs most often in southern China and Southeast Asia. Rarely have any cases been reported in western culture. The average age of patients with Koro syndrome is thirty-two. It is seen both in men who are married and men who are single. Personality characteristics of most of these men reveal that they are shy, self-effacing, nervous, and endowed with only limited intelligence. Most of the men are troubled by sexual deprivation and lack confidence in their sexual abilities.

The symptoms of this syndrome are fascinating. The patients are generally so convinced that their penis is disappearing that they hold it in their hand to keep it from vanishing. They are afraid to let go. Each episode of this anxiety attack usually lasts several hours, although prolonged attacks, lasting up to two days, have been reported. Most of the attacks occur at night when the men are thinking about sex.

The syndrome has been called Koro because in Malay, *koro* means "head of a turtle," and some perceive a similarity between the head of a turtle and the head of the penis.

In fact, there have been no documented cases of the penis shrinking away. Men who believe their penis is shrinking would do well to get on the scale and check for weight gain.

WILL THE PENIS BREAK?

Most men (and women) are startled to learn that the penis can "fracture." How does this happen, since there is no bone in the human penis such as exists in the whale, walrus, and dog? It is due to the rigidity of the penis when erect. The erectile tissue is encased in a very tough covering, and as the erectile compartments fill with blood this strong tissue becomes tightly stretched. Excessive pressure applied to this tough outer cover of the erection compartments will cause a tear. This tear allows blood from the erection compartment to escape, causing immediate swelling, pain, and bruising of the penis. Cases of fracture of the penis have been reported when a male, during vigorous vaginal insertion, misdirects the penis and it strikes the pelvic bone of the female. Fracture of the penis has also been reported during intercourse when the female is in the superior position. During vigorous thrusting her weight may be accidentally displaced to create a shearing force on the lining of the erectile compartments, resulting in a tear.

The penis may be fractured at times other than during sexual activity. On a hot July night in Richmond, Virginia, a forty-one-year-old white male, wearing sunglasses and with a gold chain around his neck, came to the emergency room with a towel in front of his Bermuda shorts. He related the following story. He was in a hotel room with his girlfriend. A disturbing breeze was wafting across the bed, which was adjacent to the window. Despite the fact he was near the height of foreplay, he went to the window and using both hands, pulled it down vigorously. He did not realize that his erect penis extended across the sill. He felt excruciating pain, followed immediately by swelling and discoloration of the skin. He took a cab to the emergency room, with his girlfriend in tow. In addition to the embarrassment of relating his story to the emergency room physician, he had the difficult task of phoning his wife to advise her he would be having surgery.

A fractured penis will usually bring the patient immediately to the emergency room. Often he will come in with a towel over his genitalia and in obvious pain. While some mild cases of a fractured penis may respond to conservative management without surgery, most urologists prefer operating to reduce the risk of scar tissue and the impotence that could result.

WOMEN'S ISSUES:
BOTH SEXES NEED TO UNDERSTAND

27

WOMEN:
WHAT YOU SHOULD KNOW ABOUT MEN WHO SUFFER FROM IMPOTENCE

Women have the understanding of the heart, which is better than that of the head.

—Author Unknown

Key Points:

- Impotence may be psychologically devastating for the male.
- A woman who understands the thoughts and feelings of the impotent male can be very supportive.
- A look into the male psyche may afford women a whole new perspective.

It may be difficult for the female partner of an impotent male to relate to the depth of despair felt by a male who cannot perform. It is almost impossible for the female to realize the degree of fear that the male has when his sexual performance is inadequate. If a female doesn't have an orgasm during every sexual encounter, she probably isn't alarmed. She generally attributes her inability to achieve orgasm to just not being in the mood. But if a male doesn't have an erection, he generally regards it as a disaster. For impotence means more than simply not being able to achieve an erection. It represents the destruction of a man's self-image. His self-confidence and self-respect dwindle. And if he cannot achieve an erection on repeated occasions and thus fails his female partner, she may become sexually unresponsive. The male then begins to complain that his partner is frigid and not interested in sexual activity, and a vicious circle is created.

A male's inadequate sexual performance affects many areas of his life. On the job he may be less effective because of his preoccupation with his sexual inadequacy. At home he may be depressed and short-tempered. His wife or female partner may become increasingly dissatisfied, and it becomes more and more likely that the relationship will break up. The divorce rate in this country is soaring, and one of the reasons most often cited is lack of sexual satisfaction at home.

It is unfortunate but true that the quality of the sexual lives of most men and women is not as high as it should be. Interviews with couples who are apparently happily married, who are financially secure, and who have never openly spoken of divorce reveal that from a sexual standpoint, many are lonely, disappointed, frustrated, and emotionally unsatisfied.

Surveys on sources of sexual conflict in marriage are very revealing. Most men believe that their marital sexual relations are too infrequent. Most women desire longer foreplay and believe that coitus itself is too brief. Most men want their wives to participate more actively in sexual relations, and many wives are displeased with their husbands' sexual manner or technique. Most women also desire more postcoital affection than they presently receive. Finally, most couples have conflicting attitudes about engaging in oral sex.

It is apparent that many couples find their sexual relationships less than ideal. This rocky foundation provides a natural setting for the development of sexual dysfunction.

In men love-inadequacy is increasing to an alarming degree, and impotence has come to be a disorder associated with modern civilization. Every impotent man forms the nucleus of a love tragedy, for impotence makes marriage impossible or may be the cause of an ill-fated one. It also undermines the health of the women, and has an equally pernicious effect on the mental lives of both husbands and wives.

This statement aptly describing the damaging effect of male sexual problems on modern society was written more than seventy years ago by a physician named Wilhelm Stekel.

Discussions with impotent patients provide a great deal of insight into how sexual difficulties affect their everyday lives. Long-imprisoned thoughts are suddenly released. It is easy to discern the mental and emotional relief that a male gains by being able to reveal a problem that has too long been contained. The following comments are indicative of the depth of discomfort that many men experience.

1. Do you think about your sexual problem often?

"It is with me all the time. I cannot shake it. When getting ready for bed it bothers me the most. I would like to try sex but I know there is no use."

"How can you forget about it? Everything you see in the movies or on television has something to do with sex. Every novel I seem to read describes sexual encounters. You go to a party and all the guests are talking about sexual conquests or telling jokes with sexual connotations."

"The problem is always on my mind except while I am concentrating at work. And even that has become more difficult. There are many young secretaries with tight skirts and loose blouses and when I see them I think about how nice it would be to be able to have intercourse. I am single and I guess I am lucky that I don't have a woman who I have to satisfy, though I would like to if I could."

"I don't think there is a day that goes by that I don't wish that I was able to have an erection. My wife and I don't talk about it and I have never discussed it with my friend, but it is on my mind. I haven't had intercourse in two years and I felt by now I would be used to it and it wouldn't bother me. But it does."

2. Has your sexual problem affected your self-image?

"Very definitely! I am forty-two years old and never felt this would happen to me. I don't feel like a complete man. When you can't satisfy your wife, how can you satisfy yourself?"

"I always wondered what it would be like to be without a penis.

Now I know. It's there but it only hangs and doesn't seem to be useful for any purpose except going to the bathroom. Every time I void I take it into my hand and am reminded that I am not normal."

"I've lost confidence. My wife says it doesn't matter, but I don't think she respects me as much anymore. There is no reason my teenage children should know about the problem, but I really wonder if they do. I'm sure my wife hasn't told them, but somehow I think they must know."

"You know the old saying about who wears the pants in the family. I still make the major decisions but wonder if I really have the right to do so. After all, I don't meet all my responsibilities as a man at home."

3. Does your wife or female partner understand the problem?

"She knows there is something wrong but isn't certain what. We still try to have relations but it doesn't seem to work. Sometimes she seems satisfied but I don't know why she would be."

"My wife fully understands my difficulty. We even had sexual counseling. At first she thought I had another woman, but fortunately this idea has been cleared up. Things are better than they were. I now satisfy her with masturbation."

"My wife doesn't understand and doesn't care. One night she told me not to start something I couldn't finish and I haven't tried since. . . . I've thought about trying sex with another woman, but I don't think I would be any more successful."

4. Has your inability to function sexually affected your daily life?

"I'm depressed. At first I only seemed to be troubled at night. It seemed that I would lie awake for hours thinking about what I couldn't do. Now, I cannot concentrate on my work. I seem to spend more time trying to do things."

"I work on an assembly line and I've got plenty of time for free thought. My job is mechanical and very boring. Not one day passes that I don't think about my problem in one way or another. It is taking me longer to do things than before."

"Nothing is like it used to be. I don't sleep as well, eat as well, or work as well."

"I am sixty-two years old, single, and have met many interesting women. Unfortunately any attempt I have had at sexual activity has been a failure. I am disappointed and distressed. I have noticed that following unsuccessful encounters I tend to overeat, which has resulted in my being overweight, which aggravates the arthritis in my knees. When I gain weight I then become more disappointed with myself. It is a vicious circle and a no-win situation."

5. Have you ever sought advice or thought about seeking advice from a friend?

"Are you kidding? I wouldn't let anyone know about this. The closest I got was once telling a joke about an impotent man. I thought that might open a discussion, but my friend only laughed and said, 'I'm sure glad I don't have that problem.' I wished I had never told the joke."

"It's funny that you mention it. My closest friend and I discuss financial matters all the time and we even know each other's salary. But I would never tell him I couldn't get an erection."

"My friend told me he was having a problem with sex. I never would have brought it up first. We had a long talk and both decided we were just getting older."

6. What would it mean to you to be able to function normally again?

"A whole new life."

"It would make me very happy and I know my wife would be pleased."

"I suppose it would mean a great deal, but I've just about given up hope."

"They say the greatest things in life are free. But now I find that even trying to have sex again is going to cost me money."

"What good am I this way?"

"I would like to say I could take it or leave it. But truthfully, I'd be a lot happier man if I were normal again."

A common complaint of impotent patients is that their partner doesn't understand the depth of their frustration, disappointment, anxiety, and fear. One of the most often heard statements from the male is something like "She says it is not really important if I can't get an erection—she still loves me" or "she says an erection isn't necessary to satisfy her."

These statements, which are intended to be helpful and supportive, may actually intensify an impotent male's frustration. Many men really don't believe their partner's comments. They simply can't conceive that their being unable to perform sexually isn't important and necessary to the relationship. In some instances, downplaying the importance of an erection sends a message to the impotent male that his partner is treating the problem too lightly. There is a danger when an impotent male's partner seems to simply accept the problem and not offer any support. The impotent male feels that the matter is unimportant to his partner, and so he is shut out from any discussion of his own feelings.

While most women are supportive of their partners, they may not appreciate the emotional impact that impotence has on a male. An analogy may be helpful. If a man cannot achieve an erection in order to satisfy his partner or himself, it in some ways is the equivalent of having lost the penis. It is a form of mental disfigurement and alteration of self-image.

28

THE EFFECTS OF IMPOTENCE ON THE FEMALE

No man is an island....
—*John Donne*

> **Key Points:**
>
> - Women can experience a whole range of feelings when their partner has erectile difficulties, including self-doubt and self-blame. As long as blame is in the relationship, the partners cannot move forward toward sexual health.
> - When there is sexual dysfunction, the quality of the relationship with the partner is tested and called into question.
> - Whenever there is sexual dysfunction, there are also opportunities for greater communication between partners.

When a woman's sexual partner experiences impotence, either a brief episode or a prolonged problem, she becomes an involved, even if unwilling, partner in the problem. Just as a man can have a variety of emotional and behavioral reactions to impotence, so can a woman. Many reactions that women have are similar to those of men. Impotence in a partner in a male couple will see the same reactions. It is understandable that circumstances that affect the intimacy of a relationship will elicit similar emotional and behavioral responses regardless of the sex of the partners.

Nancy was thirty-eight, divorced, and in love with her new boyfriend, Sam. She had always been cautious about "letting go" during sex, and rarely had an orgasm with a partner. That changed when she met Sam, a forty-five-year-old man in the process of divorce. Did he turn her on! The only problem was that Sam's erections were unpredictable. At times Sam had wonderful erections, while at other times he just lost them—at the worst moment! Nancy felt awful for him at first, but later began to doubt herself. Was she doing something wrong and turning off her new lover? She thought that she was too enthusiastic during sex and needed to tone down. Nancy even wondered if her old fears about commitment were unconsciously surfacing and making Sam anxious. Maybe she was getting old and Sam couldn't avoid noticing. Nancy didn't know what to do to help Sam or change things back to the way they were early in their relationship. She felt lost.

As we think about Nancy and her response to Sam's erectile difficulty, her experience and her emotional reactions are quite common. All of us assume that whatever happens to us is in a sense superimposed onto our basic personality, and we react accordingly. Our reactions to life circumstances are therefore in part determined by personality variables, the real situation, and our learning and experiential history. In a sense, many of our reactions are also determined by what we have told ourselves about what happened to us. This sounds like a commonsense observation. However, when it comes to matters of intimacy and sexuality, reason and common sense are often the first victims of worry. Strong, and at times irrational, emotions can take over fairly quickly. Before we know it, anxiety can snowball and the problem can be out of control. It is a valuable lesson to realize that what we tell ourselves about problems colors our responses to them. Correcting our thinking plays a great part in treatment, adaptation, and recovery in the future.

WHAT HAPPENS? IT DEPENDS!

What are some of the effects of impotence on female partners? As for men, the answer for women is "It depends." It depends on a number of factors. We saw some of them in Nancy's reaction to her boyfriend's episodic impotence. The factors that can determine a woman's response to her partner's erectile difficulties include the personality style, sexual knowledge, and experience level of the woman; her expectations about the nature of sexual intimacy; the attitude and understanding of the woman about her own sexuality; the importance of sexual intercourse to the woman's interior self and external social life; the connection the woman sees between romance, intimacy, and intercourse; the importance of sexual pleasure in the woman's life; the circumstances under which the impotence occurs; the nature, quality, and history of the relationship; the frequency and possible cause of the erectile failure; and other stresses and events going on in the woman's life.

The list covers many areas in a woman's psychological and interpersonal life, and it is easy to see that the reaction to impotence will vary from woman to woman depending on circumstances. For example, the reaction of a woman to the sexual failure of a partner in a casual episode of "recreational" sex, a "one-night stand," might be very different from that of the female partner in an ongoing relationship. The sexual failure of a casual partner can be chalked up to experience, rationalized as "his problem" (maybe), and the woman may get on with her life. Impotence in an ongoing relationship is bound to bring up serious questions: Is there something wrong with us? Where are we going with this relationship? Do you still love me?

Different still can be the woman's reaction in a marriage or long-term committed relationship. Impotence in marital and long-term committed relationships can raise the same questions just mentioned, but there is also an added dimension. These relationships by their very nature are complicated by an "A to Z" sharing that goes on in daily life together. For better or worse, multiple demands of daily living influence the environment in which a couple's sexual life exists. Therefore, when erectile difficulties occur in marriage and in long-term committed couples, there can be a ripple effect that goes beyond the bedroom and influences other segments of their lives together. Their responses will in part be determined by the characteristic way they communicate, negotiate, and solve issues that face them.

Couples can differ dramatically in the way they cope with adversity. Some partners react with characteristic avoidance of discussing the problem, hoping it will go away, and choose to live with denial and tension. Other women and their partners will confer and agree on a solution that works for both of them. When it comes to dealing with a sexual problem like impotence, partners need to be emotionally supportive and resourceful in their adaptation to the sexual difficulty and to its solution. Partners who suffer in silence ignore an opportunity for potential growth, for each can gain by facing the question of what to do about their commonly shared sexual problem.

As an example of a coping strategy, it might sound strange, but many couples who have a deep and caring relationship adjust to medically or physically related impotence by avoiding sexual situations. Some woman abstain from sex in an attempt at being supportive, or as a way to avoid overt conflict, or even to avoid making their partner suffer shame or guilt. Sometimes even when these reactions are pointed out to couples they do not feel they are avoiding dealing with the problem, but instead choosing to be close in nonsexual ways. After all, it is their relationship and it is their right to be as sexual as they please. Students of Freud often joke that "sometimes a cigar is just a cigar." In the case of certain couples who deal with impotence by choosing to be nonsexual, "sometimes denial is not denial," but rather an adaptation to which both partners agree. On the other hand, therapists might label these same coping behaviors as dysfunctional in couples who typically avoid difficulties by refusing to acknowledge or discuss them.

THE WAY SOME WOMEN RESPOND

Women have various responses to their partner's erectile difficulties. Initially, a woman might be supportive and show concern or simply ignore the problem. Over time, negative reactions, such as anger and resentment, might surface that can be directed either at the partner or herself. Certain questions might arise, such as "Is he having an affair?" or "Is he considering a break-up or a divorce?" or "Is there something wrong with me?" or even "Could he be gay?"

It is not uncommon for some women in these circumstances to cope with their frustration with fantasies of former or potential lovers, or even entertaining notions of leaving their partners. However, the thought of leaving may cause fears of separation and anxiety about the future. As a result of all these emotions and inner thoughts, a woman may experience significant performance anxiety about sex, which may only serve to compound her partner's erectile problems.

While this description of the possible reactions of women to their partner's erectile difficulties is not definitive, clinical experience shows that most women respond in a fashion that includes some of these examples. As an example of how a woman's reaction may develop and influence either the progression or the resolution of her partner's erectile difficulty, let us explore the response that involves blame.

Blame may be directed either at the situation, at the partner, or at oneself. The *situation* can sometimes be blamed for the partner's sexual difficulties and can indeed be a true cause. For example, having sex under adverse circumstances can contribute to development of the problem. However, one must be careful not to place the sole blame on the circumstances and thus avoid looking into other potential causes of erectile difficulties.

Blaming the *partner* is also common: "It is his problem, not mine." This statement is erroneous because there are no uninvolved partners in a consensual sexual relationship. Every sexual partner is involved at the most elementary level, simply because he or she is there. Moreover, blaming the partner can lead to unintended effects, such as avoiding sex. While for a woman retreating from sexual contact can be a way of avoiding sexual frustration, for her partner it risks increasing his anxiety about performance. Understandably, a woman might feel justified in avoiding sex, but avoidance does not lead to improvement, especially if it is accompanied by any demonstration of anger or resentment.

Self-blame might be a woman's most common reaction. We are aware that many women tend to blame themselves for their partner's erectile difficulties. The reason for this is twofold: Women are raised in our culture to be introspective and sensitive to their role in contributing to the quality of a relationship. In addition, our culture tends to encourage us to strive for perfection . When we combine the female sensitivity to quality relationships with a tendency toward perfectionism, we have a recipe for development of self-blame whenever relationship problems occur. Given the power of this combination of factors, it is not a great reach for a woman to engage in self-blame when her partner experiences erectile failure.

Sexual self-blame often takes the form of seeing oneself as not being good enough. Insecurities about a "deficient body" (breasts, hips, thighs, hairstyles . . .) surface, accompanied by such thoughts as "If only I had a better body, he would be more turned on and not lose his erection." Women's perceived physical imperfection is illustrated by the title of a paper that was presented at a meeting of sex therapists: "Breasts Come in Two Sizes: Too Large and Too Small." It is easy to see how a woman who has an impotent sex partner can set herself up for a cycle of self-blame.

Self-blame can in turn lead a woman to withhold herself sexually. By doing so, she not only harms herself, but also deprives her partner of an opportunity to improve his sexual functioning. She then risks contributing to his performance anxiety and his own sexual withdrawal. As with many concerns in life, the truth of the matter for the couple may lie somewhere in between the reality of the problem and their worry about it. Often it is only through careful private sharing or through couples therapy that these concerns are properly put into perspective for the betterment of the sexual relationship.

This analysis of self-blame explores the wide range of women's emotional response to a partner's erectile failure. Rather than provide fuel for both further and future problems for the partners, these emotional reactions can be seen in a positive sense. A woman's emotional reaction in these circumstances can serve to illuminate the nature of the problem and how it ties into the relationship as a whole. It is also a reminder of how fragile feminine feelings are when it comes to being a caring and actively involved sexual partner. Like many other life problems that partners must face, sexual dysfunction can serve as an occasion to bring the couple together to seek a way of overcoming the difficulty and achieving greater intimacy.

SHARING THE PROBLEM WITH OTHERS: TO TELL OR NOT TO TELL

In general, women tend to share their concerns and relate their feelings to others much more easily than men. But what about sharing sexual concerns? With whom and how? When the problem is her partner's erectile difficulties, a woman may view sharing these concerns as a boundary violation in the relationship. Some partners would even consider sharing "personal couple secrets" a betrayal, and such sharing could result in arguments and further sexual problems and alienation. The degree to which boundaries are a concern often depends on the quality of the overall relationship. Where mutual respect, trust, and freedom are couple values, the concerns for privacy are usually discussed and agreed upon. If there is sharing with others, it is usually with informed consent. For other couples, tensions rise when the male has a domineering style and forbids the woman from acting freely.

The importance of boundary issues thus varies from couple to couple and from topic to topic. What is important and confidential to one partner may be considered minor to the other. An example of extreme openness is reflected in the invisible loyalties a woman may have to her family of origin. Such loyalties make her feel guilty for not telling her mother (or sister, or other family intimate) what is happening. "Of course I told my mother that Harry has been having trouble getting it up! She's my mother! I can [must] tell her anything [everything]!" Harry then has to face his in-laws on Sunday afternoons feeling angry, under a cloud, and "impotent," while his wife may feel no sense of conflict. Obviously, loyalty conflicts can be the basis of many sexual complaints, as both a cause of the problem and as a variable that maintains it.

SHIFTS IN THE BALANCE OF THE RELATIONSHIP

When a man has erection difficulties there can be a shift in the dynamics in the relationship. As we mentioned in the previous chapter, a man can lose self-confidence because of his sexual problems and may consciously or unconsciously place himself in a more dependent position with his partner. This is not to imply that he was in control to begin with, for the relationship may have been quite balanced. Many couples can handle this usually temporary shift in the dynamics of their system. However, such a shift usually affects both partners. If a woman depends on her partner for much of her self-esteem and validation, both as a woman and as a sexual person, then his inability to have an erection places her at risk. She may ask, "If I no longer depend on him for intimacy, pleasure, and sexual satisfaction, what is going to happen to me?" Her self-esteem and integrity can be threatened. Matters can become worse if her reemerging need to be dependent on him fuels his growing anxiety about erectile failure. His own dependency on her may cause him even greater discomfort. From this scenario we can see how the notions of both anticipatory anxiety and performance anxiety become shared problems of the couple. They can interfere with the sexual functioning of either the man or the woman.

CAN THEY TALK?

The woman's response to her partner's erectile problems is also influenced by the communication style and problem-solving abilities of the couple. We will come back to this again in Chapter 40, but it is worth mentioning here. Partners tend to deal with issues in a relationship in a way that has been characteristic for them over the time they have been together. Even if an attempt at effectively communicating is unsuccessful, the ineffective pattern tends to be repeated unless one of the partners changes his or her style of relating. Thus, if the relationship is characterized by casting blame, withdrawing, engaging in hostile and passive-aggressive maneuvers, or sabotaging as a way of punishing the partner, then sexual difficulties can bring out all the worst in how a couple deals with intimacy issues. Matters only deteriorate.

As another way of handling things, some couples refuse to deal with the sexual issues and suffer in silence, drifting further apart sexually. Some therapists regard a couple's quietly drifting apart as a "collusion of silence." In other words, "If you don't say anything about the situation, neither will I." This "collusion" is a more destructive type of denial than that of the couple we referred to earlier who desire to support each other in their silence. Once again, we bring our usual way of relating and usual problem-solving capacities to our sexual life. How a woman deals with her partner's impotence will be influenced by these factors, both in the positive and negative sense. To be effective, communication about sexual matters needs to be sensitive, nonblaming, and respectful. Then the real work begins. It can be done. Unfortunately, most men are reluctant to initiate this work and, once again, depend on the woman to take up the burden and responsibility of prompting the move toward sexual health. A woman's work is never done!

29

FEMALE SEXUAL DYSFUNCTIONS AND THEIR EFFECT ON IMPOTENCE

Men always want to be a woman's first love; women have a more subtle instinct: What they like is to be a man's last romance.

—*Author unknown*

Key Points:

- There is a delicate interplay between sexual partners that influences their response to each other.
- A woman's sexual dysfunction may affect her partner's ability to have an erection.
- Sexual problems can both develop from and can impact the interpersonal and emotional aspects of a relationship.
- Female sexual dysfunctions include the inhibition of sexual desire, arousal, and orgasm. In some cases, this may stem from an aversion to sexual contact.
- Complaints of painful intercourse may suggest conditions of vaginismus and vulvodynia.
- Sexual trauma at any age can be a later cause of sexual complaints.

WHAT MEN NEED TO KNOW ABOUT WOMEN

Tom and Ellen were married for five years before the first of their two children was born. Their sex life had been open and carefree in the pre-child years of their marriage. Tom always wanted sex more frequently, but when they did have intercourse, it was generally satisfactory. Things seemed to change after the birth of their second child. Ellen just seemed to lose interest in sex. Nothing seemed to turn her on anymore. She denied being depressed. She still loved Tom. She even told her best friend that she could not care less if she ever had sex again.

Tom was frustrated. Not only did Ellen show no desire for sex, he could not get her aroused. Their usual ways of lovemaking were just flat. Tom couldn't remember the last time he'd "made her come." Tom began to doubt his own sexual performance and desirability. Perhaps he just could not please Ellen anymore. Even his erections were not what they had been. In fact, on several occasions, he had trouble "getting it up" with Ellen, even though he had been thinking about having sex with her for days. His desire for Ellen began to fade. He began to feel old. Tom began to understand why some men have affairs. He was embarrassed to mention this situation to his friends. He believed that only women were close enough to their friends for that kind of talk. Except for sex, he and Ellen had a happy, functioning family. Tom thought that Ellen must know how he felt. He wondered if he should say something to her?

The story of Tom and Ellen and their combined problems is not unique. Men may feel they have enough of a problem understanding their own sexual functioning. But men also need to understand women's sexuality and sexual functioning. Without this understanding, their own potency can be affected. Achieving this level of awareness about women is complicated, because men typically do not think in relational terms when it comes to the physical aspects of sexual performance. They may see it as their "job" to get an erection and that's it. What many men fail to understand is that the sexual responses of their partner can have an impact on their own functioning. We have already discussed in other chapters that erections are the result of a sufficient amount of physical and psychological arousal. A number of factors can inhibit a man's sexual arousal, including factors that affect his partner. There is a delicate interplay between sexual partners, with each capable of influencing the other's sexual response. Up to this point we have focused on the problems of men. It is time to focus on the female partners. Women can also experience a number of sexual difficulties and dysfunctions, and they can directly affect male erectile functioning.

How common are sexual complaints among the general population? It is difficult to say. The results of studies vary, and are at best suggestive, not truly indicative, of what many people really experience in their sex lives. (For example, early estimates by sex researchers Masters and Johnson were that 50 percent of marriages had significant sexual problems.)

While erectile failure in men is a sexual dysfunction that cannot be ignored, there are many other problems and difficulties that couples have about sex that can by themselves cause even more conflict, unhappiness, and lack of sexual satisfaction than true sexual dysfunctions such as impotence or a woman's inability to achieve orgasm. A study that reflects this was reported in the *New England Journal of Medicine*. Researchers interviewed one hundred "happily married" couples, 80 percent of whom said they felt their sexual relationship was satisfactory. Some interesting results were found upon further questioning. The women in the survey reported a 63 percent rate of actual sexual dysfunction in the areas of arousal or orgasm. When asked about sexual difficulties that were not truly dysfunctional in nature, such as partner disagreements about sex, 77 percent of the women had complaints. Furthermore, the degree of overall sexual dissatisfaction was more related to the number of difficulties the partners had in dealing with sex than to the number of diagnosable sexual dysfunctions. As we mentioned, statistics in studies may vary, and we can question the sample of people who were interviewed in this study. But what is strongly suggested is the importance of the interplay between partners in both establishing sexual satisfaction and in contributing to each other's sexual difficulties. Partners can and do affect one another sexually, whether their problems reflect difficulties in relating to one another sexually or are true sexual dysfunction.

What are these common difficulties that affect the quality of sexual functioning and sexual satisfaction in a relationship? The range is broad, but therapists frequently encounter complaints and disagreements between sexual partners in areas that usually reflect differences in levels of desire, attitudes about sexual practices, and sexual expectations. Disagreements most commonly heard are about the timing of sex, levels of sexual interest and frequency, what sexual behaviors are acceptable, foreplay, and what partners consider to be sexual turn-ons and turn-offs.

Readers can add to this list from issues in their own experience. The point is that regularly experiencing such difficulties can affect the overall quality of the sexual relationship. Continued negative interpersonal feedback in these disputed areas can lead to the development of further sexual difficulties and even to sexual dysfunctions.

Sexual problems and difficulties reflect the interpersonal and the emotional aspects of the sexual relationship. They often arise from a combination of educational deficits, psychological problems, inhibitions, and interpersonal conflicts. Many of these difficulties reflect the *emotional or feeling tone* of the relationship, which in turn affects the couple's perception of the quality of their sexual relationship. While many sexual difficulties are situational and may be related to the hectic modern lifestyle, others stem from general sexual misinformation and ongoing inadequate communication.

Sexual dysfunctions are diagnosed conditions that represent an impairment that goes beyond common sexual difficulties. Sexual dysfunctions in women (and men) can be either lifelong (since the beginning of a person's sexual functioning) or acquired over time after a period of "normal" functioning. They can exist in a general way (that is, not limited to specific types of stimulation, situations, or partners) or be specific to the situation or set of circumstances. Dysfunctions can also be due to medical conditions such as illness or medication side effects. They can be chiefly related to psychological causes or a combination of psychological and physical conditions.

Psychological causes can play a large role in contributing to the onset, recurrence, severity, and maintenance of sexual dysfunction in women. Other factors contributing to the presence of a sexual dysfunction include specific variables in cultural, ethnic, religious, gender, age, and social background that might influence levels of sexual desire, attitudes about sexual performance, and the importance of adequate sexual satisfaction. Regardless of what may be the contributing causes to the sexual situation, when a woman experiences a sexual dysfunction, her partner is affected. As we have said, in a relationship, there is no such thing as an uninvolved sexual partner!

THE RANGE OF FEMALE SEXUAL DYSFUNCTION

What types of sexual dysfunctions do women experience? In many areas, women are not very different from men where sexual dysfunctions are concerned. Much of what we are about to say about female sexual disorders can apply to men as well. Men need to understand and appreciate female sexual functioning as much as their own functioning. Being a good sexual partner requires a knowledge of both male and female sexual response. In earlier chapters we described the sexual response cycle with the term DAVOS (Desire, Arousal, Vasocongestion, Orgasm, Satisfaction). Like men, women can experience sexual problems at any point in this sexual continuum. Although less frequently than men, women can even engage in compulsive sexual behavior. Woman can also experience *sexual pain disorders* that can significantly interfere with sexual enjoyment and also affect their male partner.

Keep in mind that there can be any number of contributing causes to female dysfunction, including personal history and personality factors, partner issues, and situational factors. In addressing female dysfunctions we will be speaking of persistent problems that interfere with a woman's sexual functioning and cause marked distress in her interpersonal relationships. We are not referring to occasional and passing difficulty that can be easily understood and that responds to an obvious and commonsense intervention. Nor are we talking about problems that can be directly related to a general medical condition (such as infections or surgical trauma or scarring) or to specific nonsexual psychological conditions (such as anxiety, depression, or personality problems). Keep in mind any of these female dysfunctions that we are about to describe, even in mild forms, can influence the functioning of the male partner.

Inhibition of sexual desire

A complaint involving sexual desire can represent either low (hypoactive) sexual desire or actual aversion to sex. The first complaint describes women (and men) who experience a persistent or recurrent deficiency or even absence of sexual fantasies and desire for sexual activity. Like other dysfunctions, disorders of sexual desire can extend to all forms of sexual expression or can be related to specific situations, partners, or types of sexual activity. (Some women, for example, speak of being "turned off" by oral sex or masturbation.)

Women complaining of low desire claim little or no motivation to seek sexual stimulation and do not report feeling frustrated when they are deprived of sexual contact (like Ellen saying that she couldn't care less if she ever had sex again). They may reluctantly participate in sex with their partner, but usually report only passive compliance with little or no pleasure. The frequency of sexual contact is no true measure of the presence of sexual desire problems, because many woman may engage in intercourse to attempt to meet "nonsexual" intimacy needs or because of pressure from their partner. The whole issue of sexual desire is complicated because of the subjective nature of the complaint and because of individual differences between partners about what constitutes "normal levels" of desire. Sexual desire problems may also be related to difficulties in sexual arousal and orgasm. This is an example of how a problem in one area of the sexual response cycle can affect another area. Some women also complain of reduced desire as a result of taking antidepressant medication.

Sexual aversion disorders

Some women (and men) have a persistent and extreme aversion to all or nearly all genital sexual contact with a sexual partner. The intensity of aversion goes beyond simple lack of sexual desire. The woman (or man) suffers anxiety, fear, and disgust when placed in a situation where sexual contact with a partner is expected. The degree of anxiety experienced in sexual aversion disorders varies in intensity from mild to severe. There can be panic attacks and even physical symptoms. There can also be a range in what causes the anxiety, from kissing and touching to specific aspects such as genital secretions or vaginal penetration. In some cases, women may attempt to avoid any opportunity for sexual contact by becoming overinvolved in work or family matters, or going to bed early, or neglecting their appearance so as not to appear attractive. The stress that this sexual disorder places on a relationship is significant and can certainly affect the mood and sexual functioning of the male partner. The cause of aversion disorders often is traced to psychological inhibitions or a history of sexual trauma.

Female arousal disorder

Arousal is a sexual response that follows sexual desire, but not always. An arousal disorder is a persistent inability to obtain and maintain a level of sexual excitement (including the genital lubrication-swelling response) even with what would be considered "adequate" sexual stimulation. The word "persistent" is important because this diagnosis is not describing occasional problems with sexual arousal in the female. Women with this dysfunction complain about an inability to get excited even when they want to be. This complaint can be accompanied by a lack of a subjective sense of sexual excitement and pleasure even during sexual activity. Absence of adequate arousal can result in other sexual complaints, including orgasm problems and painful intercourse. While there can be psychological causes for this dysfunction rooted in the woman herself, the partner, or the circumstances, there are legitimate medical conditions that affect a woman's level of arousal and reduce her vaginal lubrication. These include reduced hormone levels in menopausal and postmenopausal women, vaginal irritations, diabetes, effects of radiation to the pelvic area, lactation, and substance abuse. The complaint can also be present in cases of depression, obsessive-compulsive disorder, and post-traumatic stress reactions. Arousal problems are complicated conditions, and again, they can affect the sexual functioning of the male partner.

Female orgasmic disorder

Inhibited female orgasm is often a natural sequence of inhibition in sexual excitement. While there is a normal variation among women in their ability to experience orgasm, this situation refers to a delay or absence of orgasm response in women following an "adequate phase of sexual excitement." This means that the focus, intensity, and duration of stimulation during the excitement phase is considered sufficient to "trigger" an orgasmic response in a woman. Factors also to be taken into consideration include a woman's age and sexual experience. Since orgasmic response tends to increase with age, the condition may be seen more in younger and less sexually experienced women.

Some women experience orgasm difficulties after cancer surgery on the genitalia and after spinal cord injuries. Recent attention is being paid to the role of medication such as certain antianxiety and antidepressant drugs in inhibiting female (and male) orgasm. Women who develop orgasm complaints after a history of being regularly orgasmic might look to the sexual relationship for clues to their difficulties. When orgasmic disorders occur only under certain circumstances, matters of desire and arousal may need addressing.

KNOW THY BODY

The early sexual script of some women may not have exposed them to a variety of stimulation that may help them reach orgasm. Women need to learn about their bodies, and especially about what they find to be arousing and pleasurable. When you think of it, how many women teach their daughters about the importance of enjoying sexual pleasure? Not too many female readers would say that they learned from their mothers (or either parent) about the treasure of joys that their own bodies possess. Neither do many women learn at home in their formative years about the exploration and discovery of nature's gift of sexual arousal, and the joyful anticipation of bringing and sharing these gifts with future lovers. However, the world today provides women with a new chance for sensual discovery. For example, there is growing awareness and acceptance of female masturbation, and the use of sexual aids, such as a vibrator, is now openly discussed among many women. The new openness has provided avenues to enhanced sexual experience that a generation ago may not have been thinkable.

As we mentioned, there is a great range of response in women regarding their "ability" to experience orgasm. Many women who are able to experience orgasm through noncoital clitoral stimulation (e.g., masturbation) are not able to do so through intercourse. Some women who do not meet the criteria for a diagnosis of an orgasm disorder may still require assistance to explore possible psychological inhibitions or relationship problems that may be impeding orgasm. Women's orgasm is a complicated biological response, and some of the issues surrounding a woman's "right to orgasm" have many implications aside from the matter of "normal" functioning. The psychological effect of an orgasm problem in women in many ways parallels the complaints that men have about impotence. Issues of self-esteem and concerns about body image, sexual attractiveness, and the nature and future of the relationship with the sexual partner affect women with orgasm difficulties. In addition, the inability of the male to "give his partner an orgasm" presents a problem for many men.

Sexual pain disorders in women

The experience of painful intercourse is called dyspareunia. While there is some debate in the medical community about its causes, the term denotes a condition in which there is persistent genital pain during or immediately after intercourse. The pain can be superficial, as during vaginal penetration, or deep, during thrusting in intercourse. The intensity of the pain can range from mild to sharp. There are a number of psychological causes that can be related to painful intercourse, and they are often related to self-image, fear or anxiety about sex or pregnancy, religious guilt, or conflicts about the sexual partner. These women might say that they do not like sex because it hurts. For some women, a more accurate statement might be that it hurts because they do not like sex. The pain that is experienced is real. What may be at issue is the cause. Women who are coping with a psychologically based dyspareunia may be experiencing the same conflicts as men who complain of potency problems. The male and female anatomy may be different, but emotional conflicts can still cause dysfunction in both male and female genitals.

There can also be a number of physical or medical reasons why women experience dyspareunia. It is not "all in a woman's head." Unfortunately, too many women have been given this dismissive advice by well-intentioned caregivers. Among the many physical conditions related to the complaint of painful intercourse are insufficient vaginal lubrication, vaginal infections, endometriosis, changes involving weakening of the vaginal tissues, and internal pelvic adhesions related to earlier surgery.

Vaginismus

Some coital pain can be caused by an involuntary contraction of the muscles that surround the outer third of the vagina. This condition is called vaginismus. The muscle spasms interfere with vaginal penetration. Pain results when the penis meets resistance upon attempting vaginal entry. Vaginismus is often responsible for "unconsummated" marriages when the vaginal constriction does not permit intercourse to occur. The problem often has psychological components that can affect a woman in nonsexual situations: for example, the inability to use tampons or to undergo a gynecological exam. In these cases the interference can range from simple fear or anxiety about any vaginal penetration to negative attitudes about body image that result in avoidance of self-touching. If a woman has trouble touching her own body, she may be quite anxious about her partner doing the same.

Vaginismus can be present only during times of sexual intimacy and may not occur during a gynecological examination. At other times, the condition is chronic, with the woman complaining of constant general discomfort because of muscle tension and spasms in the vaginal area. The condition may develop from negative attitudes toward sex or from earlier sexual trauma (including a significantly unpleasant experience with an initial gynecological exam). Other sexual dysfunctions, such as inhibited sexual desire, can also be present concurrently with vaginismus.

Sexual trauma

Sexual trauma, especially sexual abuse, can be a critical experience for anyone. It can cause later sexual difficulties for a woman. Many women know they were abused and have clear and uninterrupted memories of the events. This knowledge is a heavy burden to bear, but it does not necessarily condemn a woman to a lifetime of sexual dysfunction.

Many women who have had earlier negative sexual experiences are able to function well sexually as adults. Other women may experience significant difficulties that may require professional therapeutic assistance. However, there is a growing concern today among therapists that people are seeing signs of sexual abuse so often that many women are being placed at risk by being told that they "must have been abused" when perhaps they were not! Far too many adult nonsexual behavioral and psychological symptoms are being blamed on earlier sexual abuse without any substantiating proof or corroboration. Interpretations that are made without the benefit of evidence to substantiate the conclusion do a tremendous disservice to the woman as well as to her mate. This is a very real problem, for to believe or presume that one was sexually abused when one was not is also significant.

Recently, the public has become aware of the controversy over what has become known as the "false memory syndrome." The whole topic of how and what we remember of past events is under intense study. Professionals are seriously divided over the issue of "true" vs. "false" memory. For example, the belief that memories of abuse are true when they are really not can victimize the woman, her family, and anyone accused of being involved in the wrongdoing. There seems in some cases to be a difference between narrative truth (the story and events as recalled by the person) and historical truth (the actual events). Women who are told that they "must have been abused" should take their time exploring the matter, and should be wary of professionals who are too quick to find all sorts of indications of early sexual abuse and jump to conclusions. This is serious business. Exploring the roots of suspected abuse is a very sensitive matter and should be treated with caution and respect. If true abuse has occurred, it can and should be properly addressed.

Vulvodynia

This is an old problem with a new name. Other terms seen in medical literature are "burning vulva syndrome" and "vulvar vestibulitis." Vulvodynia is a feeling of vaginal or vulvar burning that some women experience before, during, after, and even apart from any genital sexual activity. Many of these women come to their doctors with a complaint of vaginismus, an almost reflexive response to the anticipated pain that an attempt at intercourse would bring. The entire sexual response cycle can be affected with consequent inhibitions of desire, arousal, orgasm, and satisfaction. This can all happen because of a painful burning feeling that can be in the general area of the external genitals and near the vaginal entrance.

Sometimes the pain is localized in an area near the vaginal entrance, a "hot spot" that if touched causes sharp pain, "like a paper cut, doctor." There may also be more than one point of painful sensitivity.

The existence of and the diagnosis of vulvodynia have caused gynecologists and women patients much confusion and frustration over the years. There are times when a physical exam yields no apparent cause and some women are led to believe that it is all in their heads. But it isn't. The pain is real. Sometimes there are physical findings that suggest a number of possible infections or allergic reactions as a cause. On the other hand, some doctors believe that no specific cause or treatment has yet been found. Still, the condition truly exists and affects many women.

Treatment ranges from the application of topical creams, special soaps, and antibiotics, to low doses of antidepressants (for their ability to decrease pain at the site), to injections of specific drugs at the site of the pain, to surgical intervention that removes the inflamed and painful area of the vagina.

The sex lives of women with vulvodynia is challenged. Many experience daily pain outside of sexual contact. Other women are fine until they attempt intercourse and then are faced with the choice of interrupting sex or enduring the pain of penetration in a sincere attempt to please their partner. Another option is to avoid genital contact altogether. All are unacceptable alternatives. To endure pain robs intercourse of pleasure for both partners. To avoid sexual contact leads to interpersonal frustration and tension for the couple. Single women do not know what to do. Even if their sexual script allows other forms of sexual pleasure and release, the avoidance of intercourse usually causes frustration, especially in a new and developing relationship. In some especially strong and caring relationships, men may become overprotective of their female partners and refrain from initiating all sexual activity in order not to put pressure on the female. Again, the female's sexual problems can weigh on the male as well.

EFFECTS OF A WOMAN'S DYSFUNCTIONS ON HER PARTNER

Can a man's erections be influenced by a woman's sexual dysfunctions? Of course they can! We said earlier that in a relationship there is no such thing as an uninvolved sexual partner. In earlier chapters we discussed how a man's concern about his erections can influence how he relates to his sexual partner. The same feelings apply to the woman's reactions to her own difficulties. She is subject to many of the same anxieties, self-doubtings, and frustrations as the male, and at the same levels. She may blame herself for her problem. She may blame him. "Why can't he turn me on? It's his responsibility." Even if she does not openly blame him, he may begin to blame himself for her difficulties. Here is where the "macho" image so many men are raised with comes to the surface. "If only I were more of a man, I could get her turned on." Or again, "A man should give a woman an orgasm." "How can she enjoy sex without coming? I know I wouldn't enjoy it if I didn't come." Thoughts like these reflect the myths and misinformation that many men carry around. Thus begins male self-doubt.

Let us assume that a man wants a cooperative partner who is willing to let go and enjoy sex as much as he does. We can then explore the effects that a woman's sexual problems have on her partner. If, for example, she has a problem with desire, she may actively avoid sexual contact, or be uninvolved if they do have sex. If he is at all aware of her feelings and mood, he will get the message. If the problem lies with her arousal, he can build up his hopes, only to be disappointed by her lack of responsiveness. Orgasm problems are a bit more complicated, for she might be quite aroused, but not able to come. If he is used to the experience of knowing she has climaxed, and if it is an integral part of their lovemaking, then he most likely will notice and begin to wonder. If she rarely had an orgasm, he may not be concerned by its absence. Her level of satisfaction may or may not be dependent on whether she has an orgasm. Remember, in order for a problem to exist, it has to cause distress in the person or relationship. A problem may not be a problem unless the couple or individual defines it as one.

But how can a woman's sexual dysfunction affect a man's erection? To begin with, a man can experience a series of emotions in response to his partner's problem. He can at first be concerned, then frustrated, and perhaps later even angry. He may avoid sex in order to avoid the problem. He can even lose interest in sex with his partner. His growing indifference can lead to an increase in symptoms in his partner, as matters may get worse between them. As a result of her dysfunction(s), he can become vulnerable to all his own hang-ups about sex and pleasure. This is similar to what a man experiences when his own issues get in the way of his having an erection, even with a "sexually healthy" partner. When the female has sexual difficulties, her problems provide the fuel for him to light a fire with his problems and doubts. If he had erection problems in the past, they may return full force.

All of this anxiety about his partner's ability to function can erode a man's *desire* for his partner, and affect his level of *arousal* toward her. Even if sexual contact is initiated, he may fail to be aroused, may lose interest in her, may stop concentrating on his level of pleasure, and may experience difficulty in obtaining or maintaining an erection. A similar pattern can develop if she is having orgasm difficulties and he gives up trying to stimulate her through intercourse. This is another scenario where he can either lose his erection or even develop other male sexual problems such as premature ejaculation, or he too may have difficulty climaxing. This latter situation describes what is called retarded ejaculation, when the male fails to ejaculate even after adequate stimulation.

It is clear that some men can develop erectile and other sexual problems in response to the sexual status of their partner. Many men just feel that they have lost interest in sex because of her inability to enjoy and participate fully. A man's response to the situation will depend on a number of factors, including his age, the overall quality of the relationship, the value that is placed on sex in the relationship, the willingness of the partner to overcome the difficulty, the couple's sexual script, and a host of characteristics and attitudes that determine his sexual sense of self. The fact that a man can develop sexual problems in response to his partner's difficulties only makes more clear the need for both partners to participate in treatment if professional help is sought.

30

A NEW HORIZON:
DOES IMPOTENCE OCCUR IN FEMALES?

The man with a new idea is considered a crank until the new idea succeeds.

—*Mark Twain*

Key Points:

- Research in the area of female sexual dysfunction has lagged behind research into male sexual problems.
- There are physiological similarities in the male and female sexual response.
- Some sexual problems in women may be due to decreased blood flow to the female organs.

While the past two decades have witnessed intense laboratory and clinical efforts in the study of male sexual dysfunction, a similar level of activity in diagnosing and treating female sexual dysfunction has not occurred.

Why has the research in the area of female sexual dysfunction lagged behind? First, the funding for research in the area of female sexual dysfunction has not kept pace with the funding for investigation of male erectile insufficiency. Second, it is not as easy to record physiological sexual changes in the female as in the male.

However, enough research has been done to suggest that male and female sexual dysfunction may have a common molecular and physiological link. Traditionally, it has been felt that most cases of female sexual dysfunction were purely psychological in origin. Recall that this was also a common belief held about male impotence until the 1980s. Now, just as it is understood that most cases of male dysfunction are in part physical in origin—caused by poor blood flow—it is possible that many cases of female dysfunction may be physical in nature as well.

Drs. Irwin Goldstein and Jennifer Berman in Boston lead the way in research in this area. They have examined the prevalence of complaints of female sexual function. The complaints of females that seem to impair the ability to engage in or enjoy satisfactory sexual activity include decreased vaginal lubrication, decreased vaginal sensation, painful vaginal penetration, increased time for vaginal arousal, and difficulty in achieving clitoral orgasm or decreased clitoral sensation. Dr. Goldstein notes that surveys comparing sexual dysfunction between male and female couples reveal that while 40 percent of men may have erectile or ejaculatory problems, 63 percent of women have arousal or orgasmic dysfunction. As is the case with males, the prevalence of sexual dysfunction increases with age in females. This may be associated with the presence of vascular risk factors as well as the onset of the menopause. The presence in females of vascular risk factors such as high blood pressure, elevated cholesterol, smoking, and obesity seems to increase with the number of complaints of vaginal and clitoral dysfunction. Dr. Goldstein postulates that atherosclerotic vascular disease of the vessels supplying the vagina and the clitoris may lead to problems of "clitoral erectile insufficiency" and "vaginal engorgement insufficiency." In experiments with New Zealand white female rabbits, Dr. Goldstein has demonstrated that tissue in the female clitoris and vagina fill with blood during sexual stimulation. This is called "engorgement." Vaginal and clitoral engorgement depends on increased vaginal and clitoral blood flow (recall that the erection in the male is also due to vascular engorgement). In rabbits induced by diet to develop atherosclerosis, there was an inhibition of vaginal and clitoral engorgement.

In women, just as in men, it has been demonstrated that a chemical (nitric oxide) is necessary for sexual arousal. Nitric oxide has been isolated from tissue in the clitoris. It is possible that nitric oxide causes a clitoral erection in women just as it causes a penile erection in men. All of these findings raise the question whether sexual dysfunction in females may in part be due to problems of blood flow as has been demonstrated in males.

Unfortunately, there is only minimal research being done in the area of female dysfunction. However, it can be hoped that the climate for research in the area of female dysfunction will change just as it did for male sexual dysfunction two decades ago. It is not beyond possibility that in the future females may have oral medication to take for problems of sexual dysfunction. In fact, some doctors are already prescribing Viagra for selected female patients, based on the theory that blood flow is equally significant for female arousal. It remains to be seen how effective Viagra will be for women. The results may answer a number of questions about female sexual function. And women who have given up hope of a fulfilling sex life may be helped.

31

SELF-ASSESSMENT FOR THE FEMALE

To thine ownself be true....

—*William Shakespeare*

> **Key Point:**
>
> • The female partner of an impotent male who assesses her own thoughts and feelings will achieve a new level of understanding about their relationship.

Many women may feel that their partner's impotence is due to their own failure and assume responsibility. This can invoke many emotions, including guilt, disappointment, and feelings of inadequacy, leading some women to avoid sexual activity. Unfortunately, many men conclude that their partner's lack of interest is due to their own inability to perform. Misinterpretation of each other's feelings can aggravate the situation and lead to a vicious cycle.

Any female whose male partner is having difficulty with his sexual functioning should assess her own understanding of the specific problem as well as evaluate their relationship. The questions below, if thoughtfully answered, should provide assistance.

1. Have you and your partner openly discussed your sexual problem?
2. Did the onset of the problem coincide with an event or change in his life or in your relationship?

3. Do you know which sexual activities are most stimulating and pleasing to your partner?

4. Does your partner try to stimulate you in a way that you really enjoy?

5. What percentage of your sexual encounters leaves you sexually satisfied?

6. Do you have sexual relations more or less often than your partner would like?

7. Do you have sexual relations more or less often than you would like?

8. Does a firmly established trust exist between you and your partner?

9. Does your relationship with your partner seem to be a solid one, even though there may be a problem with his sexual functioning?

10. If your partner has attempted intercourse and been unable to penetrate because the penis was not firm enough, how did you react? Were you supportive? Silent? Negative? How might he have interpreted that reaction?

11. If your partner cannot achieve an erection sufficient to penetrate, are there other techniques he can utilize that would be sexually satisfying to you? If so, have you discussed these with him?

12. Can you think of a reason that your partner may be less interested in you?

13. Has your partner discussed the possibility of seeking help for his sexual problem?

14. Have you encouraged your partner to seek assistance?

15. Would you be willing to accompany your partner to see a physician or sex counselor?

32

ATTENTION MEN!
MENOPAUSE DOES NOT SIGNAL AN END TO WOMEN'S SEXUAL INTEREST AND SATISFACTION

An archeologist is the best husband any woman can
have: the older she gets, the more interested he is
in her.

—*Agatha Christie*

Key Points:

- Menopause in women is a hormonally induced condition.
- Physiological changes affect a woman's physical appearance and mental attitude.
- Men should realize that menopause in women does not signal the end of sexual interest.

Many men are not well informed about sexuality in the aging female. Some who themselves may be having erectile difficulties may erroneously assume that there is no point in making an effort to improve their situation, since their partner is probably no longer interested in having sex. While simple communication between the couple might resolve misconceptions, this usually does not occur. It is important that men understand what menopause is all about, and what changes it does and does not cause in females.

Technically, menopause signals the end of the traditional menstrual cycle. The age at which this occurs varies greatly but is usually between forty-five and sixty years. This is not a disease or illness but rather a part of the normal aging process. Alteration in female hormones is responsible for most of the changes that occur. These include hot flashes, a decrease in vaginal lubrication, and less distensibility of the vagina. Compare these with normal sexual changes seen in the aging male, such as a decrease in sensitivity of the penis, less forceful expulsion of semen at the time of ejaculation, reduction in the duration of ejaculation as well as the volume of the ejaculate, and a decrease in the weight of the testicles.

Menopause has been blamed for major changes in the female's emotional state, such as depression and mood swings. While menopause may be the cause to some extent, other factors may contribute, including stress, financial concerns, worries about children, use of medications, and other illnesses. The belief among many men that women who have experienced menopause can no longer enjoy sex is simply incorrect. Not only can a sexual experience be pleasurable, many women are still able to have orgasm. Men should remember that in addition to a purely sexual relationship, a feeling of intimacy and a sharing of emotions with the partner are also most important from the female perspective.

A review of data from the Masters and Johnson Institute of Reproductive Biology in St. Louis dispels the notion that senior citizens have no interest in sex. The oldest couple treated was a ninety-three-year-old male accompanied by his eighty-eight-year-old wife. At the Loyola of Chicago Sex Clinic, 20 percent of couples treated were older than sixty-five, with the oldest being an eighty-four-year-old male and his seventy-eight-year-old wife. This reinforces the concept that age is only a number.

PREVENTING PROBLEMS: WHAT YOU NEED TO KNOW

33

HOW TO PREVENT IMPOTENCE:
THE UROLOGIST'S VIEW

Although erection dysfunction increases progressively with age, it is *not* an inevitable consequence of aging. Knowledge of the risk factors can guide *prevention strategies*. . . . Lack of sexual knowledge and anxiety about sexual performance are common contributing factors to erectile dysfunction. Education and reassurance may be helpful in *preventing* the cascade into serious erectile failure. . . .

—National Institutes of Health

Key Points:

- Impotence is usually due to reduced blood flow to the penis.
- Preserving good blood flow to the penis depends, in large part, upon lifestyle changes.
- Taking steps to avoid impotence may lead to a healthy heart.

The key to *avoiding* impotence is lifestyle changes. Since many, if not most, cases of impotence because of physical problems are a result of poor blood flow to the penis, it is important to take steps to protect blood vessels. It will be apparent that many recommendations are the same as those for patients who wish to avoid heart disease. There are four factors of utmost importance: diabetes, smoking, high fat levels in the blood, and high blood pressure. The likelihood of developing impotence because of arterial factors increases with the number of those factors present. For example, diabetics who have high blood pressure and increased fat levels in the blood and are smokers are at extremely high risk.

One begins with a diet that is low in saturated fats and also sodium. Using a saltshaker should become a thing of the past. A diet rich in grain products, fresh fruits, and vegetables and high in fiber is important.

Those who smoke have a choice. Do you wish to enjoy nicotine or sex? The evidence is overwhelming that the use of tobacco causes an impairment of blood flow not only to the heart but also to the penis. Recent data suggest that these changes may not be reversible, so it is important to avoid the damage in the first place.

As is the case for people who are concerned about their cardiovascular status, some form of exercise is prudent. Moderation is appropriate. You don't have to be a marathon runner to be a marathon performer in the bedroom.

You should review with your physician any and all medications that you are taking. For example, certain of the medicines used to treat high blood pressure are less likely to cause sexual dysfunction than others. Your doctor, not you, should be in charge of making changes.

Have your blood tested for a lipid profile, including cholesterol, triglycerides, high-density lipoproteins (HDL), and low-density lipoproteins (LDL).

In essence, the predictors of poor blood flow to the heart are the same as those for poor blood flow to the penis. The truth is that most men are already aware of the changes in lifestyle that are necessary to protect the heart. But knowledge of the potential risk of heart disease has not proved to be a sufficient motivator for lifestyle changes. Perhaps fear of becoming impotent will be a stronger stimulus for change. A male may be more willing to take preventive measures to ensure the longevity of his sex life. One patient stated that he was willing to let his "little head tell my big head what to do."

The importance of a patient's emotional state and behavioral factors cannot be underestimated in preventing impotence, both its onset and its progression. Studies have shown that patients with a malignancy, cardiovascular disease, and a host of other illnesses benefit from a positive attitude. This same positive attitude can affect the erectile process. Don't underestimate it!

34

USE IT OR LOSE IT!

I do not know what the truth may be, but I will tell
the story as 'twas told to me.

—*Sir Walter Scott*

Key Points:

- Erectile tissue of the penis requires oxygen-rich blood to remain healthy.
- Oxygen-rich blood flow is maximized during an erection.
- Having frequent erections may preserve the ability to have future erections.

Is the old adage "use it or lose it" true? Or is it just a catchphrase used by males to convince females of the importance of regular sex?

Solid scientific evidence now shows that in the flaccid (nonerect) state, the penis is in a state of anoxia (low oxygen supply). In the erect state the penis is perfused with life-sustaining, oxygen-rich blood. Most people know that if the heart does not receive sufficient oxygen-rich blood, a heart attack may occur, and if the brain is not well supplied with oxygen, a stroke may follow. What they may not realize is that the penis is another organ that requires the flow of oxygen-rich blood to remain healthy.

If the erectile bodies in the penis do not receive oxygen-rich blood, then damage may occur that prevents the erection compartment from functioning properly. Specifically, the spaces that accept and store inflowing blood in order to create distention are unable to relax. Hence, a male who is experiencing erectile insufficiency should seek help sooner rather than later, not just for the pleasure intercourse may bring, but also in order to protect the erectile tissue.

It is well known that babies, as well as very old men, have nocturnal erections. Newborn males have been noted to have an erect penis even in the delivery room. In fact, erections have been observed in the fetus during ultrasound examinations. Seventy years ago, Wilhelm Stekel noted, "The capacity for erections begins on the day of birth and extinguishes with death."

One can speculate why males have nocturnal erections. Since it is clear that the erectile tissue is better oxygenated in the erect state than in the flaccid state, the nocturnal erections may be an evolutionary adaptation to keep the penis healthy and functional and hence ensure propagation of the species.

35

HOW TO PREVENT IMPOTENCE:
THE PSYCHOLOGIST'S VIEW

Sexual health is the integration of the somatic, emotional, intellectual, and social aspects of sexual well-being, in ways that are positively enriching and that enhance personality, communication, and love.
—*World Health Organization*

Key Points:

- Sexual health is an integration of mind, body, and relationships.
- How men think about their sexuality can often influence their sexual response, and can also contribute to the cause of sexual problems. Therefore what men tell themselves about sex can influence their response and level of enjoyment.
- Men need to pay attention to all of their senses during sex, and not just focus on their genitals.
- Couples will benefit from examining their sexual script and being open to exploring change.

In earlier chapters of this book we have discussed some of the psychological causes and effects of erectile difficulties in men. As we turn to the topic of psychological prevention it would be a good thing to keep in mind the lessons learned in the earlier chapters. The quest for sexual health is an integrated whole that has as its purpose making men free from many factors which can interfere with their natural functioning.

SEXUAL HEALTH IS AN INTEGRATION OF MIND, BODY, AND RELATIONSHIPS

We have made a number of observations to conclude that men, almost by nature, remain goal- and performance-oriented. Just as women in committed relationships tend to take on a disproportionate share of household and relationship responsibilities, men tend to have a need to feel that they are in control of things. Although there has been a shift in modern culture in the way of men demonstrating power and control in worldly matters, there is still an underlying understanding in men that sexual prowess is an important indicator of strength and value.

This attitude can affect a man's general sexual health as well as specific functioning like the erectile process. Men have to examine it to enjoy the freedom of healthy sexual functioning. In order to be free for something we must be free from certain restraints. We are speaking of freedom from the psychological effects on sexual functioning of fear, shame, ignorance, false beliefs, and false guilt, all of which inhibit sexual response and impair relationships. Some of these concerns can be addressed by simple education and understanding of sexual facts and accumulation of knowledge and experience. Other freedoms are attained from gaining self-awareness about how our behaviors are influenced by our thinking and attitudes. Even when a man's capacity for erections is fine, he would be well advised to pay attention to his sexual script and practice the skills that lead to ongoing sexual health.

THINKING MAKES IT SO

As long as men continue to view their sexual life as a goal-oriented experience, they may find themselves missing much of what it means to be a sexual person. As with many things in life, our emotional response to events tends to be colored as much by what we tell ourselves about it as by the actual event itself. Therapists remind us that it is not so much what happens that upsets us, but what we tell ourselves about what happened. Thus, for example, the overall emotional response to an occasional erectile difficulty will vary. If a man can tell himself that it is not the end of the world, it won't be. However, if he tells himself that it is the end of the world, then maybe it will be, and he will react with shame, disappointment, and anxiety about the future of his sex life. This is not to suggest that one should be completely unconcerned about an incidence of impotence. It's a question of the degree of the emotional response. The most prudent course is somewhere between indifferent denial and outright panic. Right thinking is a great help in preventing sexual problems. While many sex therapists will agree that a man can't will himself an erection, there is much collective wisdom in the belief that a man can think himself out of an erection.

If we put this advice about right thinking into action, we can discover a number of ways a man can help himself and not fall victim to the psychological mechanisms that can interfere with the erectile response. The following are some suggestions that will bring together many of the points we have been addressing in this book. Let them serve as helpful reminders. Be aware of what you are telling yourself about your sexual feelings and behaviors, including any list of "shoulds" that can interfere with healthy sexual functioning.

Be realistic about expectations for yourself and your partner.

Be aware of distortions in your thinking about making love and about being open to sexual pleasure.

Examine any unresolved notions about sex being bad, dirty, or sinful, and how these attitudes may reflect on your feelings about women and their enjoyment of sex.

Look for ways that you might be distracting yourself during sexual activity, and in the process reducing your arousal level.

Beware of rushing through foreplay just to get to the main event. You could be missing meaningful pleasure and arrive at attempting penetration while insufficiently aroused. In other words, enjoy the pleasures of "outercourse" before moving to intercourse.

Examine feelings about the partner that might be acting as a turn-off.

Finally, and generally, examine your sexual script for messages, attitudes, and behaviors that need attention and changing.

The above collection of pointers is not exhaustive. To younger men, who still have "automatic erections," the questions just raised might seem unnecessary. But older men know that as a man's sexual life unfolds, whether in a new relationship or in a long-standing partnership, these issues become more and more important. Good erections depend on more than just a healthy body and genital system. The whole man becomes involved in a complex interplay of thoughts, feelings, behaviors, and relationships. Prevention of erectile dysfunction over the long haul requires paying attention to these issues. How important they are in a man's life will vary from time to time and depend on any number of circumstances. But they do not go away. Erections, however, can go away. And erectile failure does get a man's attention.

JUST WHAT IS GOOD SEX?

Most men—and women—know when they have had good sex. Much of sexual experience is subjective. If we experience something as being good for us, then we are pleased and likely to repeat it. This enlightened understanding is not meant to be a way of avoiding the possibility of growth or pursuing sexual enhancement. Instead, it frees us from objectifying, measuring, and placing a priority on goals rather than pleasure and mutual enjoyment. Yet some men don't really know what they like. They can tell you the usual—and good—things, like enjoying a good erection or an explosive orgasm with a willing and responsive partner. But have these men taken time over the years to explore pleasuring, including self-pleasuring, to the point that they can identify what pleases them, using all their senses, in a sexual experience? Many men, by focusing on genital pleasure and response, have neglected to identify what is pleasing to them in other areas of lovemaking. If a man wants to retain many years of pleasurable and fulfilling sexual functioning, including good erections, he must learn to focus on nongenital sensations that he also experiences as pleasurable, and that lead to heightened desire and arousal. Remember, the road to good erectile response travels through the land of desire and arousal.

PAYING ATTENTION TO THE SENSES

If desire and arousal are key ingredients that result in the erectile response, then men are encouraged to explore what other sensations please them. We are referring to a variety of touches, smells, tastes, sounds, and visual stimuli that to them are erotic and pleasing or both. Men can do this by learning to pay attention to sensual pleasure in everyday life and not just in sexual experiences. Once again, we can appreciate that women are raised to a greater degree to appreciate bodily sensations, textures, scents, and visual scenes that are pleasing to them. In fact, young men in particular tend to make fun of such a level of sensitivity in both women and themselves. Sometimes men gain greater sensitivity through just being with a partner over a period of time, or by raising children. These same sensitivities can be applied to one's sexual awareness and enjoyment. When something is experienced as being sensual, it is taken in by the whole person. While what is sensual may not always be genital, it can be very sexual. Many readers may remember the wonderfully humorous and sexy eating scene in the film *Tom Jones*. In the film the use of food by the couple was a form of erotic play and was a prelude to their later sexual union.

The connection between desire, arousal, and the erection response becomes obvious when we consider that the nervous system is a complex feedback loop in which all sensations, including thoughts, are interrelated and processed both by the higher brain activities and reflexive responses. Thus one sensual experience can trigger another. If the sensations are interpreted as being pleasurable, so much the better. But men may not have been paying attention to what is pleasurable to them. This is especially true if a man is too busy focusing on whether his penis is hard enough in an all-out role as spectator rather than a participant. Sometimes the best way to focus on arousal is to tune in to the partner's arousal. Many men are turned on because they are aware that their partner is turned on. They use cues from her enjoyment to enhance their own arousal and maintain their erections. Boring sex can lead to a wandering mind, a loss of focus on arousal, and eventual erectile failure. Perhaps this knowledge is in some part responsible for some women faking orgasms in order to please their partner.

EFFECTIVE COMMUNICATION

For the most part, men are action- and performance-oriented. When difficulties are met, they tend to want to fix things. The emphasis while growing up male is not as oriented toward intimacy, sharing, and connecting as it is in females. The usual life experience of men means they usually come into adulthood poorly equipped to be tuned in to their female partner's emotional and intimacy issues. In addition, many men are not in touch with how they really feel or think about things. Such a low level of self-awareness leads to difficulties in communicating adequately in relationships. Over the years, and depending on circumstances, such skill deficits can contribute to a breakdown in communication, and a growing sense of frustration and even anger in either or both partners. The result can be the development of sexual problems.

Not only are some men not in touch with what turns them on, but even if they do know, they may be reluctant to share what they want with their partners. The reasons for this are many, including embarrassment and not wanting to feel like a "dirty old man" for suggesting something that may not be in the couple's usual sexual script. Men may not know what language to use in making their requests of their partner. Sensitivity counts. There is a difference in the way sexual talk is spoken by one partner and heard by the other. Couples develop their own sexual language. For example, there can be a real difference between saying (and hearing) "It really feels good being inside of you" and "I want to screw your brains out, right now!" Either comment can be just what the partner wants to hear, but which one is right for what partner, and when? How to speak about sex is a common difficulty for men and their partners. Some women do not want to hear it. Other women welcome it. Men may not understand that many women welcome specific suggestions, either because they want to be open to explore their sexual potential or they too are too embarrassed to ask. What is important in talking about sexual preferences with a partner, even in the "heat of passion," is a sense of openness to the other. This means risk for many people. It means being able to feel free from judgment, guilt, shame, or being seen as selfish by the partner.

Openness to what each partner wants to explore sexually is important, but becoming comfortable with such disclosure does not come easily for many people. For example, men may be reluctant to suggest to their partner that they watch adult videos. When VCRs first became available, the adult films tended to be male-oriented and many women did not find the contents arousing. The sexual explicitness in these videos became, for some couples, the focus of discussion of issues of erotic preference, gender sensitivity, values, and debates about exploitation of people and sex. As a result, emotions sometimes flared, judgments were made, and many couples backed away from "sharing ideas" about what might be found to be arousing. Changes are being made in adult films, perhaps in response to market demands. Sexually explicit adult films are now being produced for couples, and are now in popular use as modes of enhancement for partners to share. Self-help and educational videos have also become a popular vehicle for couples to explore sexual concerns and further enhance communication and openness. Many women were surprised that they too were sexually aroused by erotic visual stimuli. Research in human sexual response had demonstrated this pattern of arousal years ago. Men aren't the only ones who are turned on by seeing something that they label as "sexy." Sexual scripts can change as a couple become more open to understanding and trusting what is sexually pleasing to them.

The psychological prevention of impotence presents a man with a need for an ongoing awareness of how he views and experiences his being a sexual person. As a man ages, it would serve him well to understand and reevaluate the social messages he has incorporated into his thinking about sexual functioning. He must learn to place his current sexual functioning into the context of his own sexual history, his current life circumstances, including the status of his partner relationships and his general health. He must evaluate his thinking about sex to become aware of the subtle influences of male myths and unreasonable expectations. If he is experiencing medical problems or psychological conflicts that may be affecting his erectile capacity, he must attend to them. The choice is his. He can accept what he has, or he can continue to explore and enjoy his erotic potential. It is his sex life.

36

BUILDING A HEALTHY RELATIONSHIP

Sex is a force that permeates, influences and affects every act of a person's being at every moment of existence. It is not operative in one restricted area of life (that is, sexual intercourse) but it is at the core and center of our total life response.

—*Anthony Kosnick*

Key Points:

- Sexual health flourishes in healthy relationships.
- Knowing who you are in a relationship increases the chances of intimacy.
- Relationships that foster mutual respect have a better chance of staying healthy.
- "Keeping the erotic pot bubbling" opens the door for greater sexual satisfaction.
- Good sex is how you and your partner define it.
- Time, Talk, Trust, and Touch are essential ingredients in keeping partners close.

GOOD RELATIONSHIPS AREN'T ALWAYS EASY

Impotence is all about couples. Men need to understand relationship dynamics and what promotes a connection between two people. It is not surprising that men are often inarticulate when asked to describe the strengths and weaknesses of their relationship. They are often willing to settle for things just being okay! And "just settling" is what they often get. Sometimes they do not notice the difference between an "okay" relationship and a comfortable and intimate one.

Neither are many men able to describe what they could do to promote closeness. Despite good intentions, many men are not in touch with the fine points of intimate relating. Expressing emotions in their childhood home may have been discouraged or limited to angry outbursts. Such a background can leave a man with skill deficits when it comes to feeling and expressing emotions. (Of course, women can also have had poor role models at home and they also can come into a relationship with skill deficits in many areas.)

Knowing how to communicate can be difficult for some men. A husband who loves his wife might feel that he is expressing his love in his actions, for example, by helping around the house. The same man may be confused when his spouse asks if he loves her. "Of course I do. I just fixed the back door for you without having to be asked." This scenario can apply to the wife's intentions as well. Many readers will be familiar with the scene in *Fiddler on the Roof* where the husband asks his astonished wife: "Do you love me?" Here the wife's long years of devotion to husband and family may not have been seen by the man as an expression of love for him. These are very clear examples of how good intentions may not be enough to get across a message of caring. Misunderstandings can result and needless and silent drifting apart can take place. Men may find themselves asking the old question: "Just what do women want?" Poorly developed relationship skills can lead to anger and hostility. These emotions can be a prime contributor to the development of sexual problems, especially erectile difficulties. We said earlier in this book that the penis doesn't lie! Ongoing sexual health requires healthy relationships.

INTIMACY AND THE EMOTIONAL CONNECTION

The relationship, good, bad, or indifferent, is where a couple's sexuality finds its home. Many of us live out most of our sexual lives in a relationship with some partner. Partners may come and go, but we each bring ourselves and our style of relating to those sexual encounters with another person. The sexual connection can be one of passion, love, indifference, recreation, mutual consent, or even exploitation. The crucible of the sexual relationship will find sexual contact as a union of love and affection. It can also be a demonstration of a number of emotions, including joy, anger, sadness, grief, even an attempt at intense intimacy with the other in response to the fear of loss or separation. These are very common and human expressions of our sexuality. It becomes clear that sexual expression means different things at different times over the course of an intimate relationship. The quality of the sexual experience will often depend on the quality of the relationship. This relationship quality is especially important for men and their ability to obtain and maintain an erection.

Sex and marital therapist Dr. David Schnarch reminds us that many people who are married may not be emotionally connected. Getting connected is a long and ongoing task for couples, but well worth the effort. While it may be frustrating, confusing, and infuriating, it can also be joyful, satisfying, worthwhile, and growth-enhancing. A key element is finding out who we are in the relationship, both apart from and together with one another.

What does this mean? When two people become a couple, they bring together their individual selves, personal histories, personality styles and difficulties, sexual scripts, family of origin influences, expectations of relationships, goals and aspirations, as well as many attitudes and values about living life. This is a complicated mix, but it is an unavoidable part of intimate living. A sexual relationship is constantly being lived out and negotiated within this web of intersecting elements. It is easy to see that conflicts and misunderstanding in nonsexual areas will affect the quality of the sexual relationship, and vice versa.

The tendency today is for people to want to do their own thing. The term "self-actualization" has become the mantra for many people. Individuals talk about "finding themselves." We have evolved a "culture of narcissism," a "me first" mentality that leaves little room for compromise where one's rights and wishes are concerned. While self-realization and personal growth may be admirable, are they possible within a relationship? Are couples threatened when one of the partners has a different view of individual preferences than the other? Will the tension result in conflict and alienation, or even passive suffering in silence? And what about the sex life in such a relationship?

Part of the problem, and the solution, lies in how the partners view what it means to be a couple. For some, being partners means absolute fusion. The two have now become one (flesh). If their model of being a couple is one of absolute overlap with little freedom for self, then there will be problems. Too much togetherness can be smothering, just as too much distance can lead to feeling disconnected from one's partner. What is needed is a sense of balance between the drives of being an individual and the need to be together. How is this accomplished? Through a process of differentiation and gaining a healthy sense of self.

The term "differentiation" was recently reintroduced into the sex and marital therapy literature by David Schnarch to reflect the process and ability of partners to maintain a sense of self while still remaining emotionally and physically close. The more important a person becomes to us, the greater the tendency to feel swallowed up by the other. In intimate and sexual relationships, no matter how "good " they may seem, there is the chance that one or both partners will experience a discomfort or a fear of loss of self to the other or to the relationship. The reaction in a nondifferentiated spouse to feeling "trapped" will be something like the statement "I need my space." This announcement can set off alarm signals for the other partner. However, if partners have a better sense of self and each becomes more differentiated, they can risk speaking up, disagreeing, making a stand, etc., without feeling either resentful or that they now have to get out of the relationship. Of course, the partners may not feel the same need to be differentiated. That is why attempts at movement by one member can be so threatening to the sense of self of the partner.

Dave and Ann have been married for fifteen years, have three great kids, and are each satisfied with their careers. They share many interests, but lately Dave has become more involved in professional organizations related to his legal career. He already works long hours, and Ann has begun to complain that he seems more interested in his career than his family.

In fact, this is not really the case. Dave is as devoted to Ann and the kids as ever. However, he does feel that his career opportunities have allowed him to grow in areas that are different from Ann and home. He feels guilty about discussing this and fears that Ann will feel rejected. Yet he believes he is just trying to be true to his feelings and an emerging sense of self. Dave has seen resentment grow in friends who were unable to approach their spouse with similar topics. He hasn't outgrown Ann, but he feels a need to assert and define himself in the marriage in a different way than in their early years together. It is hard for Dave to put these feelings into words.

The tension between Dave and Ann has already cut into their sexual relationship. Frequency is down. Ann seems moody. Neither his desire for Ann nor his erections are what they used to be. Dave is beginning to feel resentful. If he doesn't speak up, matters will only get worse. How can he approach Ann without risking a blowup?

The story of Dave and Ann may sound familiar. They are both good people, but they are beginning to drift apart. Part of the reason that attempts at individual growth by a partner are so anxiety-producing to the other is that so much about how we feel about ourselves is dependent on how we think our partner feels about us. In other words, our identity becomes dependent on our partner. The less differentiated people are, the more dependent they will be on their partner for their own sense of self. The less-differentiated partner can become passive or even demanding whenever he or she feels threatened in the relationship. The threatened partner reflexively seeks more fusion.

Despite the fears of the loss of the sense of self, there is really less to be concerned about than one might think. Becoming differentiated really means being able to be oneself in the relationship while also being able to be close to the other. It is not running away from the relationship in a burst of individualism. It is not selfishness, but rather self-differentiation; it is knowing who one is. It actually allows for greater intimacy in the relationship. Healthy relationships require the capacity to be intimate without being overly threatened by the intimacy. This means being afraid neither of being engulfed or of being abandoned by the other. It is played out in daily living. It is also usually brought into the bedroom, where a healthy relationship can celebrate sex freely. In contrast, a strained relationship can provide the foundation for sexual difficulties, including impotence.

AGREEING ON RELATIONSHIP GOALS

In any relationship, one partner can veto participation in any task. This is especially true when it comes to making changes in existing patterns of relating and behaving. Building skills to keep an intimate relationship on track requires not only the work itself, but also knowledge and commitment to the task. One has to know what one is striving toward to appreciate what has to be done. Not every individual or couple will be willing to put forth the effort required to make needed changes. There are challenges to face. Too much neediness on the part of either partner will interfere with the balance in the relationship. Too much individualism may prevent the couple from "looking in the same direction together." But what constitutes a good relationship? Opinions vary from couple to couple. Experienced therapists would consider some of the following notions as hallmarks of a high-functioning intimate and sexual relationship.

Relationships that respect the rights of both partners tend to be ones that are:

1. *Consensual.* That is, each partner is a willing participant in the relationship, sexual and otherwise.
2. *Nonexploitive.* The relationship does not exist for, or is not maintained at, the expense of one of the partners.
3. *Honest.* There is openness and sharing between partners that is expressed in their personal and sexual life together.
4. *Mutually pleasurable.* Both the sexual and nonsexual aspects of the relationship are gratifying for both partners.
5. *Other-enriching.* The relationship, including its sexual aspect, gives expression to a genuine interest in the well-being of the partner.
6. *Self-liberating.* The relationship creates an atmosphere in which the sexual and nonsexual sharing promotes genuine growth and spontaneity.

7. *Sexually and socially responsible.* The partners are concerned about each other's sexual health and take precautions to avoid sexually transmitted diseases.

While not every couple need to have all of these characteristics, there are times when just a small change in the way a couple relates will bring great rewards.

EVERYDAY SKILLS:
KEEPING THE EROTIC POT BUBBLING

What does it mean to keep the erotic pot bubbling? It means that a couple needs to pay attention to each other and their relationship in such a way that the romantic and the erotic are not overlooked. Remember that we said earlier that modern lifestyles conspire against our sex lives. A busy schedule offers little time for being sexy. Yet, as the old song goes, "little things mean a lot." Men do not always appreciate this as well as women do. A touch, a kiss, an absentminded caress, an erotic promise such as "Not now, but just you wait until this weekend" can be a real turn-on and serve to keep the erotic aspect of a relationship going. It is important to be realistic about a busy life schedule and not set each other up for sexual frustration by developing unrealistic expectations about sex. Just as it takes two to tango, it takes both partners to keep a sexual relationship bubbling. Remember how easy it was in the early days of a relationship when both partners had sex in mind constantly? That supercharged experience was the presence of the "automatic pilot" of Mother Nature bringing two people together sexually. Unfortunately, in many relationships, the passage of time as well as daily responsibilities can weaken the flame of desire and inhibit a man's erection response. The fire hasn't gone out yet, it just needs tending.

What is being suggested about keeping the erotic pot bubbling requires accepting oneself as a sexual person, and purposefully enhancing that awareness through conscious activity. It means that sex is something to be celebrated, not to be endured. It means examining one's sexual script for any sex-negative messages or guilty attitudes that might interfere with being spontaneous about sexual matters. It means being aware of our feelings toward our partners and not letting petty differences erode the quality of shared sexual experiences. Since keeping the erotic pot bubbling requires open communication, it provides opportunities to enhance problem-solving and negotiating skills. Enhancing these skills will bear fruit beyond just the sexual aspects of the relationship as an ever-widening circle of intimacy strengthens the relationship. It may mean building new skills and overcoming old habits, such as a shyness about addressing sexually related topics. It may require reviving old behaviors that have become rusty from neglect. Many men have gotten out of the habit of being sensual and sexual, except when attempting intercourse, and have grown out of touch not only with their erotic self but with basic intimacy issues. Keeping the erotic pot bubbling may mean work, but it is pleasurable work.

As we have said, keeping the erotic pot bubbling is essential to good sexual health. The sensual attention partners pay to each other enhances sexual desire and facilitates arousal. Attention to the sensual and the erotic nurtures the couple as sexual beings, making each person more aware of himself or herself and of the partner as people capable of sexual enjoyment. It inspires sexual confidence in a man. Confidence is a great aphrodisiac. As a result of paying more attention to sex, there may be an increase in sexual fantasy during the course of a day, as both men and women will be more tuned in to the erotic in their lives. Even if the fantasies do not directly include their partner, the general desire level is increased. Some people would say they are just more "horny" and are looking forward to being sexual. In committed relationships this means seeing the partner more as an object of one's sexual desire, someone with whom one would want to share his or her sexual side. Intimacy is enhanced and a self-rewarding and sexually reinforcing environment is established. Erections flourish in such a garden. Keep it well watered.

IS THERE A RECIPE FOR GOOD SEX?

Is there a recipe for good sex? The answer is easy. Just find out what works for you and your partner. Don't let others, including "the experts," tell you what is good for you. You decide. Remember the old question of whether the glass is half empty or half full? Satisfaction in sex is greatly a matter of subjective appraisal. One way to find out what works is to ask yourself the following question: What are the ingredients that are needed to increase the chances of a mutually satisfying sexual experience happening? Take time. Talk about it. When you and your partner have figured this out, you should ask each other: What are the barriers that get in the way of having a mutually satisfying sexual experience? Do not just acknowledge these barriers, do something about them! After all, it is your sex life.

Perhaps the answers are simple and self-evident. Conversely, the answers might be quite complicated and only serve to raise more questions. That is okay, because having more questions helps define goals. But just examining these two initial questions will tell a great deal about what is going on in the relationship that either enhances or detracts from sexual satisfaction. Just saying "My erections aren't great" is not enough. Look for what contributes to the erection problem. What helps get over it? Remember the sexual response model of DAVOS? What enhances desire and arousal? What keeps arousal going? What gets in the way? Partners should not be surprised if they discover that erections sometimes take care of themselves. Spectatoring about the status of an erection (Is it hard enough yet? What is the partner thinking about it?) can actually make matters worse.

Next focus on pleasuring—each other. Again, the results might be surprising. And—this is very important—what does it take for sexual activity to be satisfying? Is it performance or pleasure? Each couple finds their way, sometimes through trial and error, and other times with a little bit of luck. If one gets lucky, enjoy it and don't downplay it as a fluke! Always have a sense of humor. And remember, for a couple in a stable relationship, there is always tomorrow. Hasten slowly. Impatience is the companion of disappointment. Stop "catastrophizing." Is it really the end of the world? Not likely. Again, there is always tomorrow. A couple will get a lot of mileage out of tomorrows, including the benefit of more satisfying sex.

THE FOUR T'S GO A LONG WAY

There are many things partners can do to enhance a relationship and provide an environment for better sexual functioning. We can bring together these elements by examining the Four T's: Time, Talk, Trust, and Touch. The four T's are key ingredients for creating an environment for satisfying sex to take place. Together, they go a long way toward ensuring a quality relationship and open the door for sexual enrichment and healthy functioning.

Any relationship needs *time* to be nurtured and flourish. One of the major complaints of couples coming to counseling is the lack of time they have together. Their daily life places many burdens on their time. Careers and families are jealous for our attention. Couples can become so disconnected that even if they have the time to be together, they do not know how to handle it. People get overextended and drift apart, and their sex lives suffer. Having time for each other is a luxury. If wanting to have a satisfying sexual relationship is a goal, then having time and taking time is a necessity! Many men seek help for erectile problems only to complain that even when they obtain the correct advice, they do not have the time to pay attention to overcoming the problem when at home.

Practice makes perfect. And practice takes time. It is his erections he is worrying about. Do the homework! The ingredient of time also means taking time with sexual activity. This means not rushing into intercourse just because the man is worried about losing a good erection. If he can get an erection in the first place, it can come back. The plumbing is working. Be patient.

The partner needs time too. Keep the overall sexual relationship alive and not just focused on the quality of the erection. A willing and cooperative partner is essential. Pay attention to her generally, not just sexually. A quiet evening or a getaway weekend can be a tonic for a tired couple.

Talk is like shared time. It opens the door to greater intimacy. Talk allows each partner room to grow. Research studies have shown that busy couples spend only a few minutes a day talking. Even then, the conversation may be about practical necessities about managing a daily life and family matters. Does the talk ever focus on the other? How are they doing, feeling about themselves? We are not suggesting heavy, in-depth, marriage-encounter communication as a steady diet. Such an ongoing examination of the state of a relationship may for some prove to be more of a burden than a blessing. Still, it is important to connect on a regular basis through talk.

Talking does foster intimacy. How many couples can talk openly about their sexual relationship and not feel threatened by the conversation? It is too easy to feel that one partner is placing demands on or blaming the other for sexual difficulties. This is especially true when it comes to erection problems. Associations of blame, guilt, and even fear of infidelity or abandonment are common. Partners need to reassure each other that they are each involved in the sexual problem. There can be no room in a healthy relationship for a comment like "It is your problem, you fix it." The rejection that would follow such a comment causes further alienation and continued dysfunction. Talk requires facing the negative emotions behind the rejecting statement and clearing up that issue before moving on to the sexual complaint. While couples do present themselves for counseling about a sexual problem, they often have to face many relationship problems that underlie the complaint before any hope of progress can be made. Remember, the penis doesn't lie. Nonsexual issues can get in the way of sex. Talk.

Trust usually grows with time and talk. Enduring relationships are based on trust. Trust is also the basis for feeling comfortable with one another during sex. Trust eliminates the fear of ridicule and rejection and allows one to relax in the presence of the other. Trust is essential in a caring sexual relationship. As mentioned in an earlier chapter, trusting each other is more than not worrying about infidelity. It also speaks to a level of comfort with the other. Trust comes from an abiding sense that each partner is committed to the other's well-being. This doesn't mean that partners cannot disagree with each other about important issues. It does mean that no matter what stand one takes, the position is respected. Trust inspires confidence in being supported by the partner. Sexual confidence flourishes in a trusting relationship.

Touch—and response to being touched— is part of being human. We are, after all, raised and cuddled from infancy with the loving and attentive touch of parents and family. Studies show clearly that babies who do not receive the human comfort of loving touch fail to thrive. Adults also need and respond to touch. The affectionate touch between partners, both outside and inside the bedroom, is an important part of life together.

Many women who seek counseling complain that their partners pay little attention to them during a given day. These same women are surprised when they are approached by some "stranger" in bed when the lights go out at night. As far as the woman is concerned, there has been no preparation for intimacy. Here is an example of where some men really don't get it. Not only do these men not bother to touch their partners in nonsexual ways and in nonsexual situations, but they are puzzled when their partners complain when they do touch them in bed. If these men had paid attention to the need for touch in the process of keeping the erotic pot bubbling, they might be pleasantly surprised once the lights go out.

Some men (and couples) are not comfortable with touch because they have become "rusty" from lack of practice. That's right. Some people need practice to appreciate the pleasure that comes from giving and receiving touch. This is especially true when it comes to receiving an erotic touch from a partner. Many men tend to focus on the genitals as a sole target of receiving pleasurable sexual sensations. Not that there is anything wrong with that. They might, however, be pleasantly surprised to experience the stirring of genital arousal from nongenital stimulation by their partner.

Tuning in to the pleasures of touch is all part of the overall sexual enhancement that comes from being open to and practicing paying attention to our senses.

We have discussed the importance of the four ingredients of Time, Talk, Trust, and Touch in enhancing and maintaining a healthy relationship. Together, the Four T's help keep the erotic pot bubbling. When paid attention to, these ingredients provide an ongoing and ever-growing foundation for healthy relating and an environment for open, honest, and satisfying sex.

37

WHAT THE FEMALE PARTNER CAN DO TO HELP THE IMPOTENT MALE

It is better to avert a malady with care than to use physic after it has appeared.

—*Shao Tze*

Key Points:

- It is helpful if females appreciate the level of frustration and inadequacy felt by their impotent partner.
- Assessing the situation honestly will lead to better understanding.
- Impotent men who have supportive partners have a higher and faster rate of recovery.

Every female should understand that when a male cannot achieve an erection and have successful intercourse, it is a catastrophe for him. Because he has performed inadequately, his ego is shattered. He may feel anxious that his relationship is in jeopardy. He may feel guilty that he has not satisfied his partner. As one male said after experiencing several episodes of impotence, "If I can't be right, Doctor, then I would just as well be dead."

There is no question that the greatest contribution that a female can make is to be understanding. She must understand her partner's feelings and concerns. It is helpful if she reassures him that she is acquainted with this problem, at least through reading she has done, and that she knows there is help available. She should openly discuss with him anything she can do to reduce his anxiety or to stimulate him. A remark as simple as "Let's try again later" can be very supportive. On the other hand, a female partner's negative reaction or a dismissive statement such as "Don't start something you can't finish" or "Here we go again" may be devastating to the male.

The female must determine whether there is anything in her behavior or sexual performance that is contributing to the difficulty. If her partner signifies an interest or willingness to seek professional help, she must encourage him. If the counseling requires her presence, she should be a willing participant.

A female can salvage an impotent male's ego by encouraging him to satisfy her in other ways, such as by oral or manual stimulation. If she can have an orgasm utilizing these methods, the male will not feel that he has totally failed. And if she cannot have an orgasm, it is reassuring if she tells him that her total satisfaction does not depend on having an orgasm every time, and that she does enjoy those activities of which the male is capable.

Those women who sense that their partners are simply bored with their sexual relationship should try a new approach. Few women will seriously condone a relationship with another women, but many would be willing to introduce a change in their pattern of sexual activity by utilizing different forms of stimulation, such as oral sex, or by trying new positions.

The most common position for sexual intercourse in the United States is the so-called missionary position, in which the female lies on her back and the male is on top, facing her. In this position the male can easily control the rate of thrusting. Some men who are having difficulty achieving a good erection report that they can insert the partially erect penis more easily in this position. However, the male-superior position has several disadvantages, which include rapid ejaculation by many men because of vigorous thrusting and maximum penile stimulation.

Most American couples will sometimes use the female-superior position. This permits the female more control over the rate and depth of penile penetration of the vagina and allows the woman to take a more active role during intercourse. This position is often recommended by sex therapists for women who are having difficulty achieving orgasm.

The third most commonly used position in this country is probably side-to-side. Many men report that they can control ejaculation best in this position.

The rear-entry position has several variations. Both partners may be lying on their sides, or the woman may be bending over or perhaps leaning on her elbows and knees. Some couples do not approve of this position, since there is no face-to-face contact, which they feel diminishes intimacy. Also, many women complain that this position permits little clitoral stimulation. However, the clitoris can be stimulated manually if necessary.

There are numerous other coital positions, including penetration while both partners are sitting or standing. Couples should realize that no one position is either "normal" or "abnormal." However, whatever positions are used should be acceptable to both partners.

An older couple should increase the length of foreplay. With age, simple touching, caressing, and holding each other increase in importance. Older men may not ejaculate, and a woman should not force the issue, for her partner may still derive great pleasure from intercourse. Appropriate support and encouragement may prevent a problem that occurs occasionally from becoming chronic. Such support from his partner will encourage the impotent male to seek help. This in turn will help preserve the relationship.

38

CAN IMPOTENCE BE PREVENTED WHEN A PATIENT IS TREATED FOR PROSTATE CANCER?

Luck can be assisted. It is not all chance with the wise.
—*Balthasar Gracián*

Key Points:

- Prostate cancer is the most common malignancy in men in the United States.
- Curative treatment may result in erectile insufficiency, but a male's primary goal should be elimination of the malignancy.

Cancer of the prostate is the most common malignancy (excluding skin cancer) in men in the United States. A new case is diagnosed every two and a half minutes, with a death occurring from this disease every thirteen and a half minutes.

With the advent of the PSA (prostatic specific antigen) blood test, more and more men are being diagnosed with prostate cancer. The disease is being detected and treated at an earlier age, potentially reducing the death rate. Because one of the potential side effects of treatment for prostate cancer is erectile insufficiency, an increasing number of men—and their partners—are affected.

There are three major goals when treating patients for prostate cancer. The most important is to remove or eradicate all malignant cells. The second is to try to preserve urinary control. The third is to try to preserve erectile ability.

The two standard treatments available to cure prostate cancer that has not spread are removal of the prostate gland (radical prostatectomy) and radiation therapy either from a machine (external voltage) or from radioactive seeds implanted into the gland (brachytherapy). More recently a technique to freeze the prostate and eradicate the malignant cells (cryosurgery) has appeared. All of these treatments carry a risk of impotence.

Most urologists will recommend a radical prostatectomy if the malignancy is confined to the prostate gland and the patient is in reasonable medical condition. Prior to 1982, patients were likely to be impotent following radical removal of the prostate gland. In April of that year, Dr. Patrick C. Walsh of Johns Hopkins University performed the first successful "nerve-sparing radical prostatectomy." After considerable work in the anatomy laboratory, Dr. Walsh was able to identify the nerves supplying the erectile tissue of the penis and devised a technique that permitted preservation of the nerve supply.

Despite the important contribution of nerve-sparing radical prostatectomy, not all men will be potent following surgery. One of the best predictors of postoperative sexual function is the degree of preoperative potency. Patients who have other illnesses such as cardiovascular disease, hypertension, and diabetes are less likely to recover potency than men who are otherwise in good health. Patients who are cigarette smokers and consequently have impaired blood flow to the penis might also be expected to demonstrate a lower rate of sexual preservation.

The use of radiation therapy to treat prostate cancer is becoming more and more commonplace. It is very appealing to many patients who wish to avoid a surgical procedure. Many patients erroneously believe that if they choose radiation therapy they are guaranteed preservation of erectile ability. Unfortunately, this is not the case. Impotence can develop following external voltage radiation or the implantation of radioactive seeds in the prostate.

The use of cryosurgery to freeze the prostate gland in order to eradicate cancer has been reintroduced to the medical community recently. Like all treatment modalities, this form of treatment has advantages and disadvantages. However, long-term survival data are lacking and patients should understand that almost all men will be impotent after this treatment. Some patients will recover their function over time, but there is no guarantee.

It must be remembered that many men have lost their sexual potency prior to receiving treatment for prostate cancer. Clearly it is unlikely that these individuals would experience erectile ability after treatment.

Whatever treatment a patient chooses, he should be psychologically prepared for the fact that he may not have a return of sexual potency. However, as unpleasant as this is, treatment will usually add a number of years to his life.

An important new concept has arisen concerning a method to preserve erectile ability following treatment for prostate cancer, whether by surgery, radiation therapy, or cryosurgery. Patients who utilize self-administered penile injections (see Chapter 13) in the postoperative period experience a higher rate of return of erectile ability. This is most likely due to increased oxygenation of the erectile tissue. Patients generally start pharmacological therapy, or use of a vacuum constriction device, one to three months after treatment for prostate cancer. A newer technique, involving placement of medication in the tip of the penis, is also available, but its effectiveness in restoring potency is unknown. Similarly, the role of Viagra in preserving potency after treatment for prostate cancer is yet to be determined.

MOVING TOWARD
SEXUAL HEALTH

39

WHY IMPOTENT MEN DON'T RECEIVE ADVICE

I am busy meddling as always, but I am slowing
down a little bit as I read that Socrates gave advice to
everybody in Athens and they finally poisoned him.
—*Rose Kennedy*

Key Points:

- It takes courage for a male to seek help for impotence.
- Many physicians are either too embarrassed to discuss problems of
  sexuality with their patients or lack training to do so helpfully.
- Many patients are disappointed with what they perceive to be
  inadequate advice from their doctors.

It takes a certain amount of courage for an impotent male to seek professional advice. Unfortunately, there is still a stigma in the minds of many people when it comes to sexual matters. This problem is magnified because it is not only the patient who is uncertain how to address the issue. Studies have shown that most family physicians and primary care providers do not include a sexual history as part of a comprehensive initial evaluation of a new patient. Yet, these same studies indicate that the overwhelming majority of patients wish that the topic had been addressed. This is particularly true for those patients who are having sexual difficulties.

Why has a sexual history not become a standard part of a complete medical history? One reason is the carryover of the old taboo about discussing sexual problems with anyone. Another reason is that many physicians never received formal teaching during the course of their medical training. The good news is that many medical schools now include this important area as part of their core curriculum. Unfortunately, not all do.

However, the medical profession has in a sense been forced by the media to confront problems of sexuality. Many magazines, newspapers, and radio and television shows deserve credit for addressing problems of human sexuality forthrightly and in a professional manner. In many instances, the public is a step ahead of health care providers in learning about new advances in the sexual field.

The failure of physicians to counsel patients is unfortunately not limited to the sexual field. The Centers for Disease Control and Prevention concluded that many physicians fail to use office visits as an opportunity to convey important information on a topic as important as heart health. Despite the enormous impact of heart disease in our society, many doctors fail to offer basic advice to their patients about the importance of diet, exercise, weight reduction, and stopping smoking. Such advice would also help preserve potency.

The problem of the failure of physicians to counsel a captive audience (their patients) has been well documented in the case of smoking. It is estimated that 70 percent of smokers in the United States visited their physicians' offices in the past year, but only one-third of these patients were advised to stop smoking. Yet other surveys have shown that the doctor's advice is the single greatest factor in motivating a patient to discontinue the use of tobacco. It is not difficult to imagine that if a physician is reluctant or too busy to counsel a patient on the dangers of smoking, patients are not likely to receive advice on preventive measures to avoid impotence. While in some cases this might be due to a physician's being overly busy, in many instances it is because doctors doubt that they can significantly influence their patients' lifestyles through conversation. Physicians have found from experience that many patients "listen but don't hear."

But there is hope. Medical students and patients are better educated and more knowledgeable about human sexuality. The media are more attuned and willing to discuss the matter. Educational efforts such as this book are a giant step in the right direction.

40

DISCUSSING THE PROBLEM WITH YOUR PARTNER

Don't walk in front of me; I may not follow.
Don't walk behind me: I may not lead.
Walk beside me and just be my friend.

—Camus

Key Points:

- It is worth discussing your mutual sexual concerns with your partner.
- Nothing is improved by keeping silent.
- Avoid blaming one another for erectile difficulties or any other sexual problem. It is a couple issue. Both are involved.
- Be realistic about early expectations for improvement. Keep talking and keep trying.

Ken began to notice a waning of desire for sex with Barbara after only a few years of marriage. She had mild but recurrent bouts of depression that often made her "unavailable" to him sexually. At least it seemed that way to Ken. He didn't want to push her into being sexual with him, but he began to resent her apparent lack of sexual desire for him. Ken tried not to take her lack of interest personally, but she was his wife.

Ken began to find himself attracted to other women. He knew that these attractions were "understandable" when he considered the situation at home. However, he felt guilty about these temptations, even though he had never acted on them. Then his erections became totally unreliable. He found himself beginning to worry about what would happen the next time he got close to being sexual with Barbara. Yet Barbara did not seem to mind that he frequently could not perform. He became short-tempered with her. Ken was worried that matters would get worse. He knew they had to talk. But how?

By now you do not have to be told that it is not easy to talk about sex. Many men are hesitant or even afraid to share their concerns about sexual performance with their partners. Their early learning history demonstrates that admitting a sexual problem to oneself, one's friends, and especially to one's partner is no easy task. The good news is that men can learn to talk with their partners. In some cases, just talking out the problem in a trusting relationship may be all that is needed to regain lost confidence. It is certainly worth the try.

Many men would agree that talking about erectile failure during a sexual encounter is usually brief and not much help. Typical phrases said between partners might be something like "What's wrong?" or "Just don't worry about it—I don't care whether you get an erection or not, so why are you bothered by it?" Unless the conversation is continued at another time, the intended help and reassurance may miss the mark.

Dealing with a sexual problem is a risky time for both the man and his partner. You will recall from the earlier chapters on the psychological impact of impotence how much soul-searching can take place in each partner. Old insecurities and grievances can resurface as partners try to reestablish an equilibrium. If there is a history of noncommunication about important matters, then the probability of speaking about the sexual problem is remote. In fact, a collusion of silence is the way many couples avoid difficult topics, especially sexual problems.

There are guidelines that are helpful. Many are no different from when a couple is discussing any other intimate topic. They all have to do with respectful talking and listening. Male readers, pay attention to these words before you begin speaking with your partner. Slow down and think things through. To begin with, how do you view the erectile problem? What do you think is happening? Has the erectile failure been a long time in development, or do you see the impotence as situational, easily explained, and perhaps easy to correct? How disturbing is the erectile failure? Are you getting into spectatoring and becoming filled with anticipatory anxiety about sexual functioning? Is the problem reminding you of any old issues from your past? Are typical male myths about performance now contributing to your difficulty? How important do you think your problem is to your partner? Do you think it has anything to do with her? Considering these questions in advance will make any conversation considerably easier.

Sharing concerns about your partner's role in your desire and arousal levels is a touchy area. The topic is emotionally loaded. Yet remember, talking with your partner about what you like or dislike in sex need not be taken as criticism of her. Open and frank discussion about your mutual sexual script may be the road to future sexual enhancement and enrichment. Serious discussion also provides a venue for the task of "becoming oneself" within the relationship. It can be a risk well worth taking.

SOME DOS AND DON'TS

When you are ready to discuss your erectile difficulties, it would be helpful to keep the following advice in mind.

Try not to be defensive. Even though you are understandably upset with your diminished potency, admit it, and try to look at it with your partner as a shared concern. This is no time to put your whole ego on the line. Becoming defensive only distances you from your partner and puts her on the defensive too. You need to work together on this. If she refuses, then you may already have some of the answer as to why there is a difficulty in the first place.

Try not to get angry. Being angry at a time like this is obviously a roadblock to improvement. Admitting frustration is more productive! You can both relate to that.

Avoid "shoulds." Using phrases peppered with "you should" is no way to open effective lines of communication. This mistake is deadly, and not just in the area of sexual relationships. Let us look at this important issue more closely. People often find themselves feeling and reacting to their partner based on an assumption that something "should" be a certain way. These personal "shoulds" may be verbalized to the partner, or they may be kept to oneself with the partner being unaware of their being a measure of behavior. The partner is "supposed" to know what is expected of him or her anyway. It would be far better for the relationship if both partners could understand this "should" to be a personal preference rather than an absolute demand. For example, people might think that their partner "should" treat them in a certain way if he or she really loved them, or that they "should" have sex more often. Some readers might say that these statements sound perfectly reasonable, and in some matters, like fidelity, few would argue against them. However, the difficulty with this thinking for intimate relationships is that "shoulds," along with "oughts" and "musts" imply a standard that "must" be lived up to in order for the relationship to be okay. Demanding that "shoulds" be fulfilled may get in the way with effective communication and negotiating, especially in a couple's sexual life.

Actually, "shoulds" are not fair to either partner. Do not forget that many of our "shoulds" come from our own needs, backgrounds, and personal issues, be they healthy or neurotic. Our "shoulds" can place unrealistic demands on our partners (and on ourselves, as in "A good spouse or parent should . . . "). Failure to meet these expectations can serve as a basis for judging the spouse as adequate, loving, committed, etc. Finally, a person might not even be aware of the existence of his or her own "shoulds." We all have our personal list. It would be helpful to examine them.

Above all, avoid blame. Placing blame doesn't get you anywhere except to make your partner become defensive or feel guilty. There is a big difference between discussing a partner's role in the sexual difficulty and heaping all the responsibility on her or him. "If only you were . . . " You fill in the details. There may be truth in the feeling behind a critical statement, such as a reference to a serious personal problem or area of ongoing conflict. Arriving at a mutual understanding of the truth requires respect, consideration for the other, and patience in the process of getting feelings and concerns out in the open. In other words, take your time. Do not rush. The return to sexual health is too important to rush the healing process. Do be patient. Support each other.

On the other hand, some men and their partners make the mistake of taking too much time to talk about important topics. Sometimes open-ended discussions can go on and on with little resolution, and these marathons often result in growing frustration and even anger. The usual complaint after experiencing such an extended dialogue is "See, I told you we can't talk about important things without making matters worse." Keep in mind that more is gained by keeping the discussion brief and to the point than by engaging in a broad, long-winded discussion. Brief discussions keep the partners focused. They allow partners to return to the topic in the future with a sense of having been heard and a confidence that they will not be trapped in an endless list of complaints for which they may feel they have no solution. Brief talks allow partners to take more risks in being open with one another. Time between meetings allows each to collect thoughts and cool emotions. Partners can try out strategies that they have developed and can return to check them out at a future discussion. Brief discussions assist the decision-making process about how and where to proceed. They help partners to be realistic about their expectations about current and future sexual functioning.

Talking about sexual problems means calling into focus many of the issues we have previously raised about what causes erectile dysfunction in a man. Any discussion with a partner should include an honest appraisal of just what ingredients a man needs to fuel his desire and maintain arousal. The partner should be able to express the same. This discussion requires a mutual acknowledgment that each of you is a sexual person who has urges, needs, and wishes to be communicated and to be satisfied. It is not so simple as to say that one person is right in his or her wishes while the other is wrong. Since the nature of sexual relationships is so complex, many people lose sight of their right to have a reasonable goal as to what their sex lives could be. The sexual life of a couple is a continuous journey that can take many turns. People do not have to get lost along the way. Keep talking!

Once you begin talking, make it count by taking action on whatever you both decide. For example, if you feel that your hectic schedule is responsible for your sexual difficulties, you should agree to spend intimate time together that will not have sexual performance as a goal. This way, you can be together in a nondemanding, pleasurable activity that will both reduce anxiety and foster closeness. You may want to proceed slowly, in order to find a way that works for you on the journey back toward good erectile functioning. Again, busy, real-life demands may get in the way of the progress you desire. As we said earlier, when you are in a relationship, there is always tomorrow. Keep talking and keep trying. It might be the man's erection that we are focusing on, but you are in this together. There is no such thing as an uninvolved partner. Let her in on the recovery process. Then you both can celebrate success.

41

WHERE DO I GET HELP?

We must love them both—those whose opinions
we share and those whose opinions we reject. For
both have labored in the search for truth, and both
have helped us in the finding of it.

—St. Thomas Aquinas

Key Points:

- Not all physicians and therapists are comfortable giving advice about sexual matters.
- You may have to take the initiative in discussing an erection problem with a professional.
- Many mental health professionals (psychologists, sex therapists, psychiatrists) are well trained in the evaluation and treatment of sexual dysfunctions.
- Clergy may or may not be a good resource for seeking assistance with sexual complaints.
- Some professional organizations dealing with sexual sciences can be a good resource for referral to qualified professionals in the field.

Even when a man admits to himself that he has an erection problem, he is still faced with the daunting question of where to turn for help. Since the problems can be either physical or psychological, the ideal place would be a professional group or center where both physicians and mental health professionals work together on the assessment, diagnosis, and treatment of sexual disorders. While there are some centers, especially in major cities, that specialize in the treatment of sexual disorders, there is no national group that certifies such centers. The patient is left with a hit-or-miss chance of finding the right place for him to obtain help.

Ideally, all physicians and mental health professionals would be well trained in the evaluation and treatment of sexual disorders. Unfortunately, this is not the case. Physicians can order basic laboratory tests that check male hormone levels or screen for the common health problems that can interfere with potency. They can identify what medications the man may be taking that can interfere with erections. But when it comes to knowledge and attitudes about sexuality, physicians can be subject to the same biases and misconceptions as the general public. Some will make sound medical decisions, but give insufficient advice about the practical management of the sexual problem. There are times when neither the doctor nor the patient is comfortable with talking about sex.

The patient may be told that everything is fine and not to worry about being able to get an erection. For some men, this advice might be a helpful and supportive comment. For others, it may be a lost opportunity because a referral for treatment to a mental health professional may never be made. In fact, not all physicians believe in therapy for patients with sexual complaints.

What should be done? Speak up if you have sexual concerns! The doctor won't faint. The reluctance of men even to ask questions of their doctors is a reminder of the depth of the male myths about sexual functioning. Thou shalt not have any sexual problems. The myth of the perfect penis lives!

MEDICAL SPECIALISTS

Some men seek assistance from their primary physician. They may be referred to a urologist for further consultation. Or they may go directly to the urologist on their own for an evaluation. The urologist is a physician who specializes in the functioning and disorders of the urogenital system and is equipped to order the special tests needed to evaluate the medical aspects of the complaint of impotence. Once the assessment is completed and the diagnosis is made, the urologist may make treatment recommendations, which could include medication, mechanical devices, or, in some cases, surgery. These recommendations may be the most appropriate whenever physical causes for impotence are discovered. However, it is sometimes even more helpful to use an interdisciplinary approach and include a mental health professional in the treatment plan, such as a psychologist or psychiatrist who also specializes in dealing with sexual disorders.

There are times when the proper medical advice may not be enough to deal with the problem. Many men have been prescribed drugs and provided with injections that, while indicated medically, did not enhance their sex lives because the relationship with their partner was not addressed as part of treatment. It is also true that many men may have been given the proper prescription, but failed to use it. Something was missing in the connection between the man's request for assistance and his willingness to follow through on the directions. This pattern frequently happens in matters of general health. We are often given sound advice by our doctors, but do not always follow their recommendations. These same dynamics are at work when doctors give medical advice about sexual dysfunctions.

You will recall our use of the term PLISSIT in Chapter 12 to describe the levels of intervention for sexual problems. Some men only require Permission-giving, Limited Information, or Specific Suggestions to get the help they need. But when they get the advice they need, they should follow it. As with different types of aircraft, some men need a longer runway before they are ready to take off into cooperating with treatment. Ideally, a good assessment of the problem as well as of the patient's motivation for treatment should be made before a doctor suggests therapeutic intervention. Doctors can take the patient only so far along the path that leads to the return to sexual health. The real work has to be done by the patient.

MENTAL HEALTH PROFESSIONALS

Mental health professionals include licensed psychologists, psychiatrists, psychiatric social workers, and nurse clinicians who have had specific training and experience in the assessment and treatment of sexual disorders. An important criteria is that the therapists be licensed in their discipline, where they have learned the basics of evaluation and treatment of psychological and relationship problems. Look for nationally certified sex therapists and sex counselors. A certified sex therapist is usually originally trained in one of the health or mental health care specialties. There are also many fine and experienced therapists, including marital and family therapists, who, while not trained in dealing with sexual dysfunctions, may be very helpful in dealing with the relationship issues that accompany erectile difficulties.

CLERGY

Few clergy are trained to deal with sexual problems. Many clergy today are reluctant to offer more than basic general counseling and are quick to recommend a professional therapist. The clergy person may function well as a referral source to professionals trained in the human sexuality field.

As we discussed in Chapter 24, some denominations may have somewhat "sex-negative" outlooks, and congregants may be understandably reluctant to discuss sexual concerns with their clergy person. Some clergy try to mix the findings of modern psychology with "old" theology and end up with both bad psychology and bad theology. For example, to state that masturbation is a "normal" behavior but still a "sin" is not very helpful. These "double messages" can lead to confusion and mistrust. There are, however, many skilled pastoral counselors who have taken training in working with sexual problems. These pastoral counselors can address the sexual problems of a person while also providing the special comfort of a clerical presence.

WHAT TO DO, WHERE TO GO, WHAT TO ASK

If a man has concerns about physical or medical causes of his erectile difficulties, he should start with his primary care physician, a urologist, or a medically based men's health center. If the man is in a major city where there is a medical school or teaching hospital, he may be able to receive some direction from these sources. The local county medical society or the local or state psychological association may be able to provide the name of a sexuality specialist. Many hospitals also have a referral hot line that can direct potential patients to a specialist.

Many therapists who have taken training in sex therapy belong to one of several professional organizations that maintain ongoing training for its members through professional journals and conferences— for example, the Society for the Scientific Study of Sexuality (SSSS) and the Society for Sex Therapy and Research (SSTAR). Membership in a professional organization is no guarantee of professional expertise, but can reflect the therapist's special professional interest in communicating with colleagues within similar specialty areas. There are national organizations that offer certification in sexual counseling and therapy, awarded only after the candidate has met strict criteria for education, training, and clinical experience in human sexuality.

One such organization is the American Association of Sex Educators, Counselors, and Therapists (AASECT), P.O. Box 238 , Mount Vernon, IA 52314; phone 319-895-8407; fax 319-895-6203. AASECT can provide you with names of certified sexuality counselors and therapists in your area. The original disciplines of these therapists may vary—for example, from psychology to social work—but they all have met AASECT criteria before receiving certification. AASECT therapists are also required to participate in continuing education credits in order to maintain their certification.

Another organization is the American Board of Sexology (ABS), 1929 18th Street NW, Suite 1166, Washington, DC 20009, phone 202-462-2122. ABS maintains a registry of diplomates in sexology that it has certified as meeting its educational and experiential requirements. ABS is a more recent certification body and, while not as large as AASECT, does have diplomates who are also AASECT-certified.

In seeking assistance for sexual problems from a therapist, it is important to remember that there are many fine therapists who have not sought certification in sexual counseling but who are excellent clinicians and can be very helpful. Many senior-level and experienced therapists choose not to pursue certification, but are still interested in maintaining their skills through attending conferences and keeping up with the professional literature. These clinicians are available and are generally known by their colleagues. In addition, many hospitals and local and state medical and psychological societies provide information on specialists in their area. These resources are available to the general public. Spending a little bit of time locating the appropriate therapist may be a wise choice.

CONCLUDING
THOUGHTS

42

SOME GOOD NEWS:
BEING SEXUALLY ACTIVE MAY ADD YEARS TO YOUR LIFE

Winston Churchill once said, "I never say 'it gives me great pleasure' to speak to any audience because there are only a few activities from which I derive intense pleasure and speaking is not one of them." But he did use the phrase on one occasion. At the Other Club, an informal group he organized to discuss ideas and politics, a standard rite was an extemporaneous talk. From one hat a name of a member was drawn and from another a topic. Once, Churchill's name was drawn along with the subject "Sex." Churchill rose and pointing to the card began, "It gives me great pleasure . . ." and then sat down.

Key Points:

- Throughout history, sexual activity has generally been regarded as a pleasurable activity. Now scientific evidence demonstrates that it is associated with a longer life span.
- Increased longevity is also seen in women who find sexual activity fulfilling and satisfying.

Not only is sexual activity pleasurable, as noted by Churchill, it is associated with increased longevity. A study of aging and sexual activity revealed that the frequency of sexual intercourse was inversely related to mortality in men. In other words, more sexually active males had a lower death rate. Interestingly, a female's enjoyment of intercourse was related to mortality as well. The more enjoyable a woman found sex, the lower was the death rate for a given age group. The quantity of sexual activity seems more important to men, while women are more focused on quality of the relationship.

A recent study conducted in the town of Caerphilly, South Wales, and five adjacent villages examined the relationship between frequency of orgasms and mortality. Nine hundred and eighteen men between the ages of forty-five and fifty-nine years were the subjects. The results are startling. The risk of mortality was 50 percent less in males with "high orgasmic frequency." This finding weakens the view that one should refrain from frequent sexual activity in order to protect quality and quantity of life.

A closer look at the data reveals that a man's risk of death from a heart attack decreased by 36 percent if his number of orgasms reached one hundred per year. The optimist will believe that increased sexual activity confers increased longevity. The pessimist will believe the opposite—that good health permits increased sexual activity. We prefer optimism.

It is not unusual for a male patient to jokingly request a written prescription from his urologist that he can show to his wife, indicating the "need" for more sexual activity. Now, in fact, there are scientific data associating sexual activity with a healthy heart. For some men, their dream has come true.

43

CONCLUSION

The most welcome messages that humans deliver to one another often come in just three words. Think of "I Love You" or "There's No Charge" or "And in Conclusion."

—Author unknown

Impotence Is Not Inevitable.

It Is Preventable and Treatable.

Sexual Health Is Yours!

REFERENCES

"The Aging Male. Can Hormones Help?" *Harvard Men's Health Watch*, Vol. 1, No. 12 (July 1997) pp. 1–3.

Annon, J. S. *The Behavioral Treatment of Sexual Problems*. Honolulu: Enabling Systems, 1975.

Diagnostic and Statistical Manual of Mental Disorders (DSM-IV). Washington, DC: American Psychiatric Association, 1994.

Feldman, H. A., Goldstein, I., Hatzichristou, G., Krane, R. J., and McKinley, J. B. "Impotence and Its Medical and Psychosocial Correlates: Results of the Massachusetts Male Aging Study." *Journal of Urology*, Vol. 51 (January 1994), pp. 54–61.

Frank, E. "Frequency of Sexual Dysfunction in 'Normal' Couples." *New England Journal of Medicine*, Vol. 299 (1978), pp. 111–15.

Gould, L. A. "Impact of Cardiovascular Disease on Male Sexual Function." *Medical Aspects of Human Sexuality*, Vol. 23 (April 1989), pp. 24–27.

Hirsch, A. R. "Scent and Sexual Arousal: Could Fragrance Help Relieve Sexual Dysfunction?" *Medical Aspects of Human Sexuality*, Vol. 1, No. 3 (June 1998).

Hunt, M. "Sexual Behavior in the 1970's." *Playboy*, October 1973, p. 84.

Impotence. NIH Consensus Statement, Vol. 10, No. 4 (December 7–9 1992).

Johnson, J. *Disorders of Sexual Potency in the Male*. London: Pergamon, 1968.

Kinsey, A. C., Pomeroy, W. B., and Martin, C. R. *Sexual Behavior in the Human Male*. Philadelphia: Saunders, 1948.

Korenman, S. G., and Lue, T. F., *Erectile Dysfunction: Current Concepts*. Upjohn Company, 1994.

Kosnick, A. *Human Sexuality: New Directions in American Catholic Thought*. New York: Paulist Press, 1977.

Lazarus, A. A. *The Practice of Multimodal Therapy*. New York: McGraw-Hill, 1981.

Levine, S. B. "Intrapsychic and Interpersonal Aspects of Impotence: Psychogenic Erectile Dysfunction." Ch.8 in R. C. Rosen and S. R. Leiblum, *Erectile Disorders: Assessment and Treatment*. New York: Guilford Press, 1992.

Lief, H. I. "Classification of Sexual Disorders." Ch. 7 in *Sexual Problems in Medical Practice*. Monroe, Wis.: American Medical Association, 1981.

Lief, H. I. "Sexual Concerns and Difficulties and Their Treatment." Ch. 11 in *Sexual Problems in Medical Practice*. Monroe, Wis.: American Medical Association, 1981.

LoPiccolo, J. "Postmodern Sex Therapy for Erectile Failure." Ch. 7 in R. C. Rosen and S. R. Leiblum, *Erectile Disorders: Assessment and Treatment*. New York: Guilford Press, 1992.

Masters, W., and Johnson, V. *Human Sexual Inadequacy*. Boston: Little, Brown, 1970.

Masters, W., and Johnson, V. *Human Sexual Response*. Boston: Little, Brown, 1966.

McCarthy, B. W. "Treatment of Erectile Dysfunction with Single Men." Ch. 12 in R. C. Rosen and S. R. Leiblum, *Erectile Disorders: Assessment and Treatment*. New York: Guilford Press, 1992

Milsten, R. *Male Sexual Function: Myth, Fantasy and Reality*. New York: Avon Books, 1979.

Morley, J. E., et al. "Relationship of Penile Brachial Pressure Index to Myocardial Infarction and Cerebral Vascular Accidents in Older Men." *American Journal of Medicine*, Vol. 84 (March 1988), pp. 445–46.

Muller, J. E., et al. "Triggering Myocardial Infarction by Sexual Activity." *Journal of the American Medical Association*, Vol. 275, No. 18 (1996), pp. 1405–09.

Pearlman, C. E., and Kobashi, L. I. "Frequency of Intercourse in Men." *Journal of Urology*, Vol. 107 (February 1972) p. 298.

Renshaw, D. C. "Is There Sex After Menopause?" *Medical Aspects of Human Sexuality*, Vol. 1, No. 1 (February 1998), pp. 7–11.

Sarrel, L. J. & Sarrel, P. M. "Sexual Unfolding in Adolescents." In Max Sugar, ed., *Atypical Adolescence and Sexuality*. New York: W. W. Norton, 1990.

Schnarch, D. *Constructing the Sexual Crucible*. New York: W. W. Norton, 1991.

Schnarch, D. *Passionate Marriage*. New York: W. W. Norton, 1997.

Segraves, R. T., and Segraves, K. B. "Human Sexuality and Aging." *Journal of Sex Education and Therapy*, Vol. 21, No. 2 (1995), pp. 88–102.

"Sex and the Heart." *Harvard Men's Health Watch*, Vol. 3, No. 12 (July 1997), pp. 6–8.

Simon, W., and Gagnon, J. H. "Sexual Scripts: Permanence and Change." *Archives of Sexual Behavior*, Vol. 15 (1986), pp. 97–120.

Slowinski, J. W. "Religious Influence on Sexual Attitudes and Functioning." In V. L. Bullough and B. Bullough, eds., *Human Sexuality: An Encyclopedia*. New York: Garland, 1994

Slowinski, J. W. "Sexual Adjustment and Religious Training: A Sex Therapist's Perspective." In Ronald M. Green, ed., *Religion and Sexual Health*. Hingham, Mass.: Kluwer Academic Publishers, 1992.

Slowinski, J. W., and Stayton, W. R., chapter editors. "Sexual Values and Moral Development." In R. T. Francoeur, ed., *Becoming a Sexual Person*. New York: Macmillan, 1991.

Slowinski, J. W., and Leiblum, S. R., chapter editors. "Sexual Problems and Therapies." In R. T. Francoeur, ed., *Becoming a Sexual Person*. New York: Macmillan, 1991.

Smith, G. D., Frankel, S., and Yarnel, J. "Sex and Death: Are They Related? Findings from the Caerphilly Cohort Study." *British Medical Journal*, Vol. 515 (20–27 December 1997), pp. 1641–46.

Stekel, W. *Impotence in the Male*. New York: Liveright Publishing Corporation, 1927.

Student, J. "No Sex, Please . . . We're College Graduates." *American Demographics*. February 1998, pp. 18–23.

Thomas, Laurie. Verbal communication on the "penis captivus" phenomenon.

"When Reporters Get It Wrong." *Contemporary Sexuality*, Vol. 31, No. 6 (June 1997). p. 3.

Williams, W. *It's Up to You, Sidney*. Baltimore: William & Wilkins, 1985.

Williams, W. *Rekindling Desire*. Oakland, Calif.: New Harbinger, 1988.

Zilbergeld, B. "The Man Behind the Broken Penis: Social and Psychological Determinants of Erectile Failure." Ch. 2 in R. C. Rosen and S. R. Leiblum, *Erectile Disorders: Assessment and Treatment*. New York: Guilford Press, 1992.

Zilbergeld, B. *The New Male Sexuality*. New York: Bantam Books, 1992.

INDEX